Contents

Preface iv

Acknowledgements vi

Introduction viii

SEWA Rural (Society for Education, Welfare and Action): 1985 (India) 1

Sustaining health development in Ayadaw: 1986 (Myanmar) 17

The three eras of primary health care: 1986 (Thailand) 37

Family Welfare Movement (Pembinaan Kesejahteraan Keluarga - PKK) and its achievements in national development: 1988 (Indonesia) 53

Integrated Child Development Scheme (ICDS): 1990 (India) 69

Community-based rehabilitation: Improving the quality of life of people with less ability: 1992 (Indonesia) 83

Paradigm shift through development programmes in selected villages of Haryana: Arpana Research and Charities Trust–India: 1993 (India) 97

Society for Health Education (SHE): 1996 (Maldives) 115

Mongar health services development project: 1997 (Bhutan) 125

The triumphant journey of FPA Sri Lanka: Sasakawa and beyond: 2004 (Sri Lanka) 147

International Leprosy Union (India): "Life is beautiful": 2006 (India) 171

Never give up: 2012 (Indonesia) 183

Annexes

Statutes of the Sasakawa Health Prize (as amended in January 1998) 195

Sasakawa Health Prize Guidelines (as amended in January 1998) 197

Recipients of the Sasakawa Health Prize 199

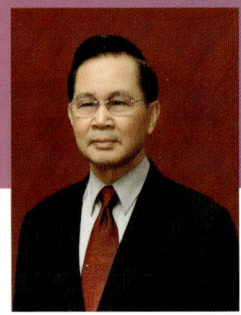

The Sasakawa Health Prize was established in 1984 on the initiative of and with generous funding from Mr Ryoichi Sasakawa, Chairman of the Japan Shipbuilding Industry Foundation and President of the Sasakawa Memorial Health Foundation.

The Sasakawa Health Prize is awarded annually to one or more individuals, government institutions or nongovernmental organizations for outstanding and innovative work in health development such as the promotion of health programmes or notable advances in primary health care. The prize is awarded at a special ceremony during the World Health Assembly and consists of a statuette and a sum of US$ 100 000.

It is a matter of great satisfaction that candidates from South-East Asia have received the prize 12 times since its inception. This is testimony to the fact that the Region is committed to the principles of egalitarianism, social justice and equity in health as enshrined in the Alma-Ata Declaration of 1978 and the ensuing Health for All movement.

This publication attempts to capture the spirit of each of these award-winning experiences. It not only presents the historical perspectives of health development in South-East Asia but also the vast repertoire of initiatives and learning that can guide us in revitalizing primary health care.

A common thread that runs through the work of all the awardees is the primacy accorded to a people-centred and holistic approach to health development. A recurring theme in the projects is the recognition of good health as an essential component of "quality of life". Another is a genuine attempt to reach out to social groups on the fringes of society. One can also discern that a large majority of these projects relied on traditional wisdom, values and beliefs, and community resources to work towards community empowerment. The spiritual ethos, volunteerism and altruism that are so integral to the culture of South-East Asia are clearly seen to be the guiding principles of these projects.

Sasakawa Health Prize:
STORIES FROM SOUTH-EAST ASIA

Preface

The experiences described in this book are an eclectic mix of health interventions and projects by government agencies, nongovernmental organizations, the community and individuals. Each of these describes the challenges that were faced, how these were overcome and the opportunities that were harnessed to achieve goals. Indeed, these are real-life examples that exemplify the challenges of intersectoral coordination and show how individuals, communities, nongovernmental organizations and governments can work together for the common purpose of improving the quality of life of the people.

It is gratifying to note that not only has the prize-winning work been sustained but also that several projects have left a lasting impact on national health policies. The write-ups contain several examples of good practices that have been adopted by national development programmes.

In addition to its archival value, it is hoped that this publication will be found useful by policy-makers, health managers, public health professionals and others to design and further strengthen their health systems using the primary healthcare approach.

Finally, I wish to express my appreciation to the many individuals who helped to research the material and draft some of the chapters and to Dr Palitha Abeykoon who served as the overall editor of this publication.

Samlee Plianbangchang

Dr Samlee Plianbangchang
Regional Director

Acknowledgements

This publication required efforts of many individuals and institutions in the South-East Asia Region, for the collection of historical information, drafting and revising chapters, undertaking reviews and providing comments. Their contributions are deeply appreciated.

The following deserve special mention for preparing the first drafts:

- **Pankaj Shah,**
Community Health and Managing Trustee
SEWA Rural, Post: Jhagadia, Dist: Bharuch,
Pin: 393 110, State: Gujarat, India

- **U Than Sein,**
Former Director, WHO South-East Asia Region
No.490, 1st Floor, Mahabandoola Road, Between 29 & 30 Street, Pabedan Township, Yangon, Myanmar

- **Amorn Nondasuta,**
Former Permanent Secretary of Health, Founder of the Primary Health Care System and President of Quality of Life Foundation in Thailand

- **Palitha Abeykoon,**
Former Director, WHO South-East Asia Region
17, Horton Towers, Colombo 8, Sri Lanka

- **Handojo Tjandrakusuma,**
Former Director of the CBR Development and Training Center (CBR-DTC) PPRBM Prof.Dr.Soeharso – YPAC Nasional
Jl.LU.Adi Sucipto KM-7 Colomadu-Solo 57176 Indonesia

- **Anne Robinson and Aruna Dayal,**
Arpana Research & Charities Trust, Madhuban, Karnal, Haryana, India

- **Asna Luthfee,**
Programme Associate, Society for Health Education, Male, Maldives

- **Sonam Ugen,**
Community Health Department,
Jigme Dorji Wangchuck National Referral Hospital (JDWNRH),
Ministry of Health, Royal Government of Bhutan

- **Sabina Omar,**
Family Planning Association of Sri Lanka, Bullers Lane, Colombo 7, Sri Lanka

- **S.D Gokhale,**
International Leprosy Union-Health Alliance, 1779/84, Gurutrayee, Near Bharat Scout Ground, Sadashiv Peth, Pune-411030, India

- **Syamsi Dhuha Foundation (SDF)**
Jl. Ir. H. Juanda 369 Komp. DDK No. 1
Bandung 40135 Indonesia

Valuable comments were provided by:

- **U Ko Ko,**
Regional Director Emeritus, World Health Organization, South-East Asia Region and formerly President of the Myanmar Academy of Medical Sciences, Yangon, Myanmar

- **U Mya Tu,**
Former Director of Health System Development, WHO South-East Asia Region and formerly Director-General of Department of Medical Research in Burma (Myanmar)

- **Agus Suwandono,**
Senior Researcher, Center for Biomedical and Basic Health Technology, National Institute of Health Research and Development (NIHRD), Ministry of Health Republic of Indonesia, Gedung 4 Labdu Lantai 6, Jl. Percetakan Negara 29, Jakarta Pusat 10560, Indonesia

- **Monirul Islam**
Director of Health Systems Development, WHO Regional Office for South-East Asia, New Delhi, India

- **Athula Kahandaliyanage**
Director of Sustainable Development and Healthy Environment, WHO Regional Office for South-East Asia, New Delhi, India

- **Secretariat of PKK**
c/o Directorate General of Rural Community Empowerment
Ministry of Home Affairs Republic of Indonesia
Jalan Raya Pasar Minggu Km 19, Jakarta Selatan, INDONESIA

The following staff members of the WHO Regional Office for South-East Asia and WHO Headquarters (in alphabetical order) provided useful technical inputs and facilitated in the collection of historical information:

- Boosaba Sanguanprasit
- Ilsa Sri Laraswati Nelwan
- Iyanthi Abeyewickreme
- Jigmi Singay
- Marie Sarah Villemin partow
- Myo Thet Htoon
- Nyo Nyo Kyaing
- Nyoman Kumara Rai

- Payden
- Prakin Suchaxaya
- Rajesh Bhatia
- Renu Garg
- Sangay Thinley
- Sara Varughese
- Sudhansh Malhotra

Editorial:

Chief Editor - Palitha Abeykoon

Editorial Coordinator - Anchalee Chamchuklin

Language Editor - Jitendra Tuli and Bandana Malhotra

Layout - Puneet Dhingra, Subhankar Bhowmik and Chander Prakash Sharma

References verification - A. K. Sharma

Special thanks to Regional Director, Dr Samlee Plianbangchang, for his inspiration and guidance.

Introduction

The Sasakawa Health Prize was established in 1984 at the initiative of and with funds provided by Mr Ryoichi Sasakawa, Chairman of the Japan Shipbuilding Industry Foundation and President of the Sasakawa Memorial Health Foundation.

The prize consists of a statuette and a sum of US$ 100 000 to be given to one or more persons, institutions or nongovernmental organizations that have accomplished outstanding innovative work in health development. The prize aims at further encouraging such work in health development, which extends far beyond the call of normal duties; it is not intended as a reward for excellent performance by a candidate of duties normally expected of an official occupying a government position or of a governmental or intergovernmental institution. The prize is awarded at a special ceremony during the World Health Assembly.

At the time the prize was established, the major criteria laid down for the assessment of the work to be recognized included the following:

(a). Contribution to the successful formulation and implementation of the national policy and strategy for Health for All by the year 2000;

(b). Promotion of and substantial achievement in advancing given health programmes, which have resulted in increasing primary health care coverage, and/or improving the quality of health care to the population, and a notable reduction in given health problems;

(c). Contribution to increased efficiency and management of health systems; policy development, health legislation and ethics, within the framework of primary health care;

(d). Innovative programmes to reach socially and geographically disadvantaged population groups;

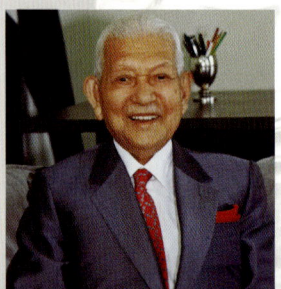

Mr. Ryoichi Sasakawa

This prize aims at appreciating accomplishments of work in the field of health development

(e). Innovative efforts to train and educate health workers in primary health care;

(f). Successful and effective efforts at involving communities in planning, managing and evaluating primary health care programmes;

(g). Development and successful application of health systems research for the advancement of primary health care.

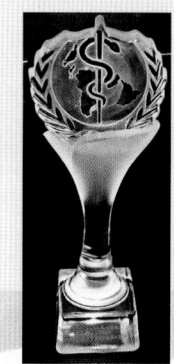

Since its inception, the prize, has been awarded to 12 winners, both individuals and institutions, from the South-East Asia Region. This is the largest number from a single Region of the World Health Organization (WHO). India and Philippines won the prize four times, the most by any one Member State, with the Indonesia ranking second (three times). Three individual winners from the Region have been honoured, personalities who have made a distinctive and outstanding contribution to health development – Dr Amorn Nondasuta, former Permanent Secretary of Health, Thailand; Professor B. N. Tandon, former Professor of Medicine at the All India Institute of Medical Sciences, New Delhi, India; and Dr Handojo Tjandrakusuma, the Founder of the Community Based Rehabilitation Development and Training Centre] from Solo, Indonesia.

This collection of Sasakawa Health Prize-winning stories from the South-East Asia Region of the World Health Organization (WHO) highlights the work done by the respective institutions and individuals, which earned them this prestigious award. As one of the main objectives of the prize is to encourage the further development of such work, a brief description of the contributions that have been made by them since the time they won the award have also been included, either as an epilogue or a post script or an "afterword" in some of the stories.

The health projects and programmes described in this publication depict a wide variety of innovative and interesting initiatives, each one based on the cardinal principles and practice of primary health care. There are many lessons that could be learnt from these experiences by all the leaders and practitioners of innovative health development, particularly those in South-East Asia.

An attempt has been made to be as faithful as possible to the original submissions that were made to WHO, limiting the editing to clarify and highlight certain significant points and principles. A few of the stories have been presented in part as first person accounts as they were experienced and evolved over time.

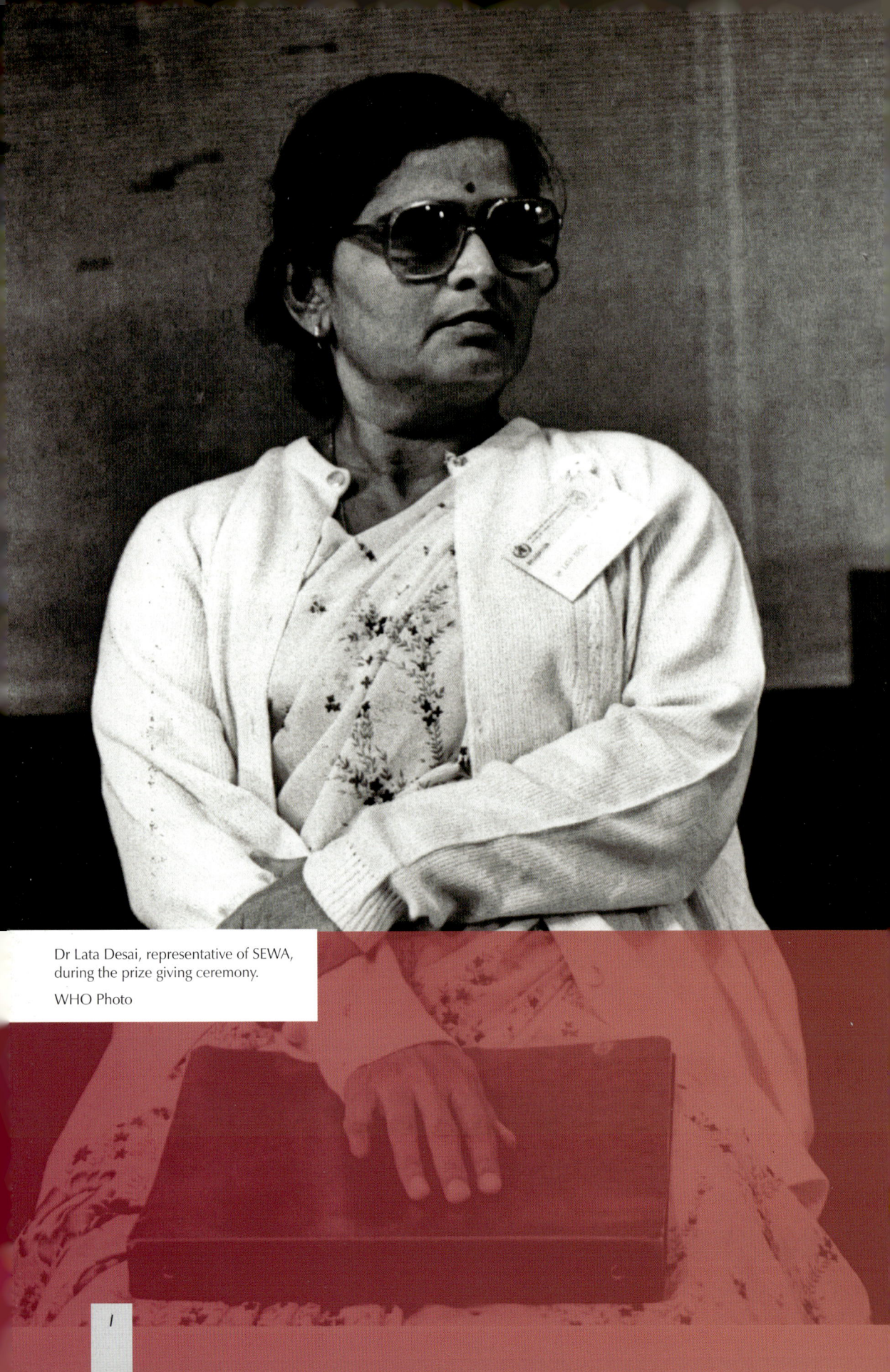

Dr Lata Desai, representative of SEWA, during the prize giving ceremony.

WHO Photo

CHAPTER **1**

1985

SEWA Rural (Society for Education, Welfare and Action), India[*]

Recipient: Sewa-Rural (society for
education, welfare and action - rural)
India

[*] The initial draft was prepared by Mrs Pankaj Shah.
Community Health and Managing Trustee
SEWA Rural, Post: Jhagadia, Dist: Bharuch, Pin: 393 110,
State: Gujarat, India

SEWA Rural is a voluntary organization involved in heath and development activities since 1980 in the rural tribal area of Jhagadia in south Gujarat

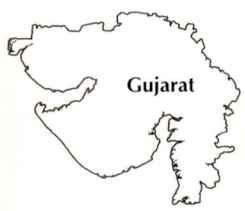

SEWA Rural endeavours to reach out and assist the poorest of the poor through various health and development programmes based on community needs and available human resources

1. Introduction

In 1984, the Society for Education, Welfare and Action (SEWA Rural) had just completed four years of work among the rural, tribal and poor communities of south Gujarat in western India when nominations were sent for the Sasakawa Prize for the year 1985. SEWA Rural has now completed three decades of its community health and development work. This article recapitulates what was done by SEWA Rural in the early 1980s to earn the prestigious prize and how subsequent work evolved and developed.

SEWA Rural is a voluntary organization involved in heath and development activities since 1980 in the rural tribal area of Jhagadia in south Gujarat. It was started by a group of young professionals educated in India and abroad, and based on the ideas and ideals of Swami Vivekananda and Gandhiji. Over the years, many like-minded youngsters have joined the organization.

SEWA Rural endeavours to reach out and assist the poorest of the poor through various health and development programmes based on community needs and available human resources. It seeks to ensure that values are preserved and self-development, in the broader sense, is achieved simultaneously of those involved in the work. The focus of all programmes has been vulnerable members of the family, i.e. women, children and the elderly, and the poor sections of society.

In all the activities, an attempt is made to incorporate as well as balance three basic principles: social service, a scientific approach and spiritual outlook. Activities include a community hospital, community health project, training centre in health, comprehensive eye care programme, community-based rehabilitation programme for the blind, vocational training centre, women's development and empowerment programme (now under an independent organization, Sharada Mahila Vikas Society). The organization believes in taking assistance from all sectors of civil society, which include the local community, individual well-wishers and donors, voluntary organizations, government and private industries, charitable trusts, academic institutions and foreign agencies. Their whole-hearted support and encouragement have ensured that the fruits of development and growth in society ultimately reach the marginalized and underserved sections of society, i.e. women, tribals and the poor.

2. The beginning of the community health project

SEWA Rural started in 1980 with a small hospital given by a local community. The organization felt that curative support, the main strength of the initial group, would be essential for primary health work. After working in the community hospital for two years, building a reasonable community rapport and assessing the baseline health status, the community health project was launched in 10 villages in October 1982. Oxfam (UK) and Community Aid Abroad (Australia) provided financial assistance. To avoid duplication of services at the community level, SEWA Rural approached state health officials with a request that the responsibility for village-level workers (community health volunteers [CHVs], traditional birth attendants [TBAs] and *anganwadi* workers [AWWs]) from selected villages be entrusted to SEWA Rural. Besides supporting and monitoring village-based workers and further building community rapport, a weekly mobile dispensary was also started in these villages so that minor ailments could be treated in the village itself. Meanwhile, the joint United States Agency for International Development (USAID)/Government of India's Private Voluntary Organisation for Health (PVOH) scheme was announced in 1983 to support voluntary organizations working for community health. Over the next five years, SEWA Rural gradually expanded the scope and coverage of its community health project to cover about 40 villages and a population of 40 000 under this scheme.

SEWA Rural gradually expanded the scope and coverage of its community health project to cover about 40 villages and a population of 40 000 under the scheme

Dr Lata Desai, representative of SEWA, addressing the 38th World Health Assembly.
WHO Photo

The focus of all programmes has been vulnerable members of the family, i.e. women, children and the elderly, and the poor sections of society

SEWA RURAL
(SOCIETY FOR EDUCATION, WELFARE AND ACTION),
INDIA: 1985 (INDIA)

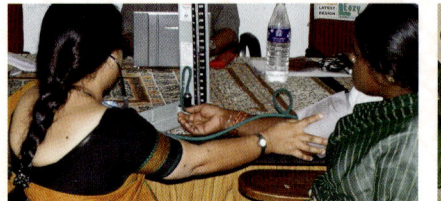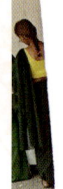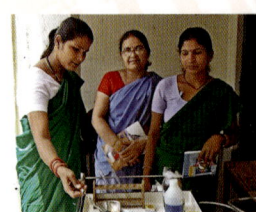

3. Key innovations leading to candidature for the Sasakawa Health Prize

3.1 Maternal services in the community health project

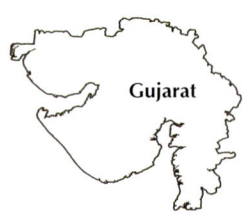

This component is given high importance as it has an impact on infant, perinatal and maternal mortality. Care is provided through the cooperative and collective efforts of CHVs, TBAs, AWWs, multipurpose health workers female (MPHW – female/FHW). The latter take active responsibility for providing this service in their respective target areas at the village level. FHWs make repeated visits to the home of every pregnant woman and provide a standard package of antenatal care (Inj. tetanus toxoid, tablet folic acid, medical examination, referral and health education).

Maternal services are given high importance as it has an impact on infant, perinatal and maternal mortality

It was observed that TBAs were not actively involved in antenatal care. They were called only at the time of the delivery. Thus CHVs, who also lived and worked in the village, maintained the register of the expectant mother, which was passed on to the FHW during the biweekly meeting at the hospital or the latter's field visit to the village. Following training, TBAs are now involved in providing antenatal care.

In rural India, most of the deliveries are conducted at home by a local birth attendant. It is not possible, desirable or necessary to replace them. What is needed is to train them in scientific techniques. Those TBAs who were not trained in the government primary health centre were provided training through the use of posters, slides and other audiovisual aids; those already trained were given refresher training. Four sessions were organized in less than a year. Training continued during the field and mobile visits to the villages. The self-esteem of the TBAs improved and they were given importance in the organization as a result of their involvement and cooperation. Their performance also improved markedly.

Presterilized delivery pack and its distribution system: The concept of a pre-packed delivery pack is not new. However, there were two areas of innovation – how the delivery pack reaches the beneficiary and how monitoring is done to ensure that it had been used properly. Expectant women are given a prepacked delivery pack by the FHW during the later part of their pregnancy (either eighth or ninth month). The woman is given necessary relevant health education and also told about the importance about the delivery pack, which she is supposed to give to the TBA at the time of delivery. The health education component of the delivery pack is given a lot of importance. As a result, the mother, mother-in-law, neighbours as well as other pregnant women are informed about the importance and details of the delivery pack. The TBA has been already trained to use the pack. It contains pieces of gauze, cotton, thread and antiseptic solution all wrapped in the bag, which itself can be used as a towel on which to place the boiled instruments and equipment when they are spread open at the time of delivery. The standard *dai* kit contains other instruments for conducting a safe delivery such as a bowl, a pair of scissors, etc. The TBA conducts the delivery as per the training she has received. After delivery, the empty bag is retained by the mother in her home and not taken by the TBA who conducted the delivery.

"High-risk" mother approach and antenatal week: Systematic training is given to TBAs, FHWs and other staff with the important objective of teaching them to identify "high-risk" mothers. The TBA is paid an additional honorarium even if she has to send such a mother to the hospital for delivery. This prevents TBAs from conducting abnormal deliveries at home, which may be a risk to the mother and newborn.

The programme has a second tier of a "mobile health team", which visits each village once a week to provide curative services and supervise village-level staff, among other work. Out of four weeks, one week is especially devoted to the identification and treatment of "high-risk" mothers, which is designated the "antenatal week". High-risk mothers who have already been identified by the FHW and TBA are asked to be present at the mobile medical van. The Lady Medical Officer examines these mothers and gives appropriate advice. Some of them are advised to come to the community hospital, and the others to the hospital, keeping the TBA in the picture.

> In rural India, most of the deliveries are conducted at home by a local birth attendant. It is important to train these attendants in scientific techniques

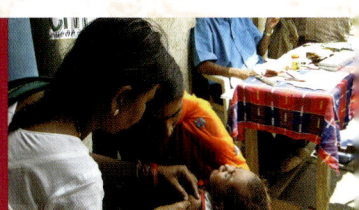

> The programme has a second tier of a "mobile health team", which visits each village once a week to provide curative services and supervise village-level staff

SEWA Rural
(Society for Education, Welfare and Action),
India: 1985 (India)

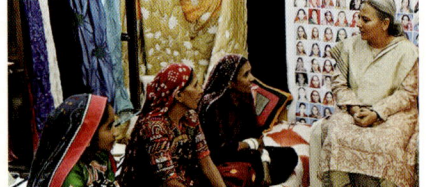 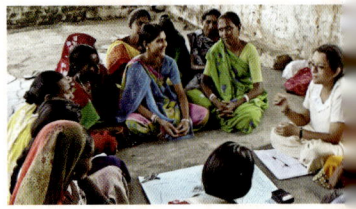

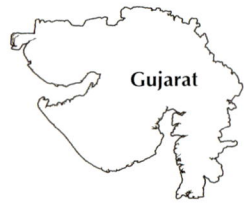
Gujarat

SEWA Rural's approach has been to work with the government in a spirit of cooperation and coordination

3.2 Community health project and government participation

Rationale: Delivering primary health care in the interior rural areas has not been an easy task. Various agencies – the government, voluntary organizations (VOs), the private sector and practitioners of indigenous systems –have all tried to tackle this problem in different ways. Each has a distinct role to play. The programme strategy needs to be formulated according to the local conditions. From the beginning, SEWA Rural's approach has been to work with the government in a spirit of cooperation and coordination. The reasons for this approach include ensuring financial support from the government for long-term sustainability, the large amount of work required to implement primary health services, ensuring replicability, creating a demand from the community through health awareness, and avoiding confusion and duplication of services.

The beginning: SEWA Rural approached the district *panchayat* and the state health directorate asking that responsibility for existing peripheral health workers (CHVs, TBAs and AWWs) be given to SEWA Rural. The workers came under the technical supervision and administrative control of SEWA Rural. A pre-test was done to assess the existing knowledge and skills of the workers, following which training was organized based on the findings. Slowly, rapport and confidence were built up with them. A unique experimental model of a collaborative partnership between a nongovernmental organization (NGO) and a government organization (GO) was launched in 1984. An area of about 40 villages with 40 000 population was handed over to SEWA Rural for total health care for five years. Of these, 21 villages would be in the first stage. SEWA Rural would be totally responsible for the health care of the people of this area. All national and state health programmes would be implemented only through SEWA Rural. All village-level health personnel (CHVs, AWWs and TBAs) would work under SEWA Rural, which would have total responsibility and power. Existing government middle-level MPHWs were given a choice; either to work under SEWA Rural on deputation or opt for a transfer to another part of the district. All existing village-level government buildings (sub-centres) would be handed over to SEWA Rural along with equipment and other fixtures. The government would financially assist SEWA Rural in paying salaries, buying medicines, etc. The organization would maintain financial and functional accountability. The district *panchayat* would appoint an evaluation committee consisting of three representatives of the district *panchayat*/state health directorates, three representatives of SEWA Rural and three members from an outside agency.

The process: Even though handing over total health care to SEWA Rural was accepted in principle, many details needed to be worked out, including the necessary government resolutions. Most of the existing middle-level health workers (MPHWs) refused to join SEWA Rural on deputation. Male MPHWs were recruited fresh and in-service training was organized. However, female MPHWs were difficult to find. SEWA Rural obtained approval as a field training centre for FHW students studying in nursing schools and recruited two qualified FHWs on deputation. Four local girls were selected by SEWA Rural and sent for the formal FHW training course. One male and one female supervisor were deputed to SEWA Rural from the government.

Though government officials at state and district levels were positive about the collaborative experiment, there was some resistance from district and block *panchayats*, as they are controlled by different political parties. Intense efforts were required to ameliorate this situation through frequent meetings and dialogue with the respective stakeholders.

3.3 Referral system

SEWA Rural was fully convinced that the community health programme needed to be backed by adequate referral support in order to boost the confidence of the community in health workers and SEWA Rural, and for the project to have better outcomes. After identifying and providing medical care to referred patients, further follow-up at the community level also formed an integral part of the referral system.

3.4 Mobilization, motivation and participation in SEWA Rural

Most government and nongovernmental programmes have the necessary ingredients for achieving the desired results. The major problem is *implementation* of the programme, and human resources are a key factor for this. Systemic efforts were made to motivate staff members at all levels for better performance and self-development.

> **Though government officials at state and district levels were positive about the collaborative experiment, there was some resistance from district and block** *panchayats*, **as they are controlled by different political parties**

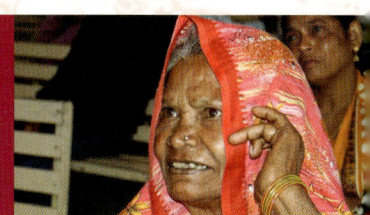

An area of about 40 villages with 40 000 population was handed over to SEWA Rural for total health care for five years

SEWA RURAL
(SOCIETY FOR EDUCATION, WELFARE AND ACTION), INDIA: 1985 (INDIA)

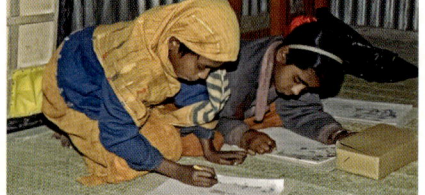
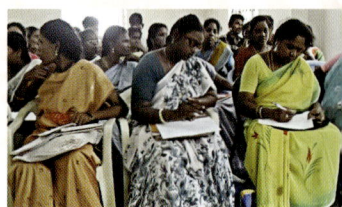

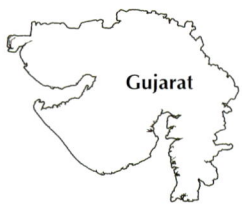
Gujarat

Over and above the fixed monthly honorarium, peripheral health workers are paid additional performance-based incentives

3.5 Encouraging peripheral health workers

Over and above the fixed monthly honorarium, peripheral health workers are paid additional performance-based incentives, e.g. a CHV is paid extra for attending educational meetings or the mobile van, helping in the detection of new tuberculosis (TB) patients, motivating people for family planning or conducting follow up. Emoluments are also given to the AWW for improving the status of high-risk children, maintaining cleanliness of the *anganwadi*, and for better attendance and adequate medical coverage of children. These workers are given importance at the mobile vans as well as at the hospital. SEWA Rural workers also try to be involved in the local festivals, customs and social gatherings along with the peripheral health workers. Thus, all efforts are made to convince the community that the peripheral-level health worker is fully backed up by SEWA Rural and is part and parcel of the team.

All peripheral health workers are encouraged and appreciated for their performance during the regular sessions at headquarters. The good work done by workers is shared with all. Their present problems and difficulties are given due attention. However, any point of criticism is discussed in person. Combined meetings with CHVs, AWWs and TBAs are organized regularly to build up team spirit and a sense of togetherness and better coordination.

Changing attitudes and creating self-confidence in the peripheral health workers is a very slow process, as they have remained neglected for many years. It requires a great deal of patience, perseverance and hard work to induce productive changes among peripheral-level village health workers who are envisaged by SEWA Rural as "change agents" of the future.

4. Epilogue

It is 25 years since SEWA Rural was awarded the Sasakawa Health Prize. Since then, there has been considerable development in its health service delivery. Other development programmes have been conducted not only in SEWA Rural but also in the larger society. These are given below.

4.1 NGO–GO collaboration for primary health care

A unique development took place following involvement of the Government of India/USAID to manage the health care of 40 villages. The Government of Gujarat handed over all existing health responsibility to SEWA Rural and transferred all their staff members (doctors, supervisors, health workers, etc.) elsewhere. Besides USAID funds for certain additional expenses, the State Government agreed to reimburse all middle-level staff-related and other routine expenditure, with SEWA Rural as a functional primary health centre during 1984–89. In spite of some limitations and difficulties, the experiment was effective, resulting in the Government of Gujarat granting formal primary health-care coverage of 40 villages (population of 40 000) to SEWA Rural for 10 years from 1989 to 1999. This was for the first time in India that the government had handed over health care and all aspects of management with 100% financial assistance.

Reviews of the community health project including NGO–GO partnership

Two reviews of the community health project were carried out by external agencies. The first covered the project period between 1984 and 1989, and the second between 1989 and 1999, when the government entrusted primary health care to SEWA Rural for a decade. Beside improvement in various health indicators and involvement of frontline workers, both studies highlighted the NGO–GO partnership.

The first review: This focused on the strengths and shortcomings of the project, and helped SEWA Rural, as well as other interested organizations and individuals, to learn. As has emerged from this study, the achievements in terms of health improvement have been significant and indicate what can possibly be achieved in other rural areas through the existing pattern of health delivery.

> It requires a great deal of patience, perseverance and hard work to induce productive changes among peripheral-level village health workers

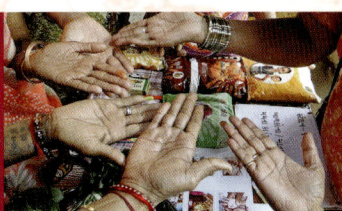

SEWA rural workers are encouraged to get involved in the local festivals, customs and social gatherings along with the peripheral health workers

SEWA Rural
(Society for Education, Welfare and Action),
India: 1985 (India)

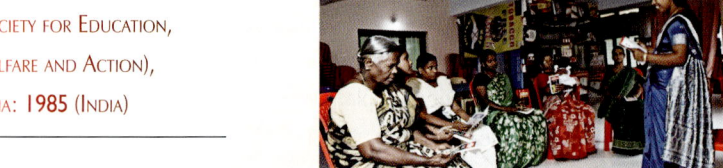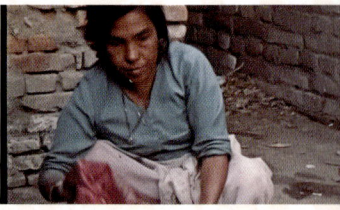

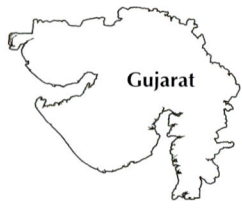

SEWA Rural experience has been an almost lone success story among a series of NGO–GO collaborations that have misfired, especially in the health sector

Impact and achievements: Health service utilization targets for Health for All (HFA) 2000 had already been achieved. In the case of many of the vital indicators too, HFA targets for 1990 had been achieved, notably the birth rate, infant mortality rate, couple protection rate, and under-five mortality rate, among others. Maternal and perinatal mortality rates remained somewhat higher as compared to HFA targets, though only maternal mortality was higher than comparable rates for Gujarat state. Measles had virtually ceased to be a killer in the project area and vitamin A deficiency in children had been controlled. Neonatal tetanus was rare as was severe childhood tuberculosis. Severe childhood malnutrition had declined, though modestly. Tuberculosis case detection was less than satisfactory, while case-holding was fairly high. Malaria continued to be a problem, though possibly less than elsewhere in the country. Definitive figures for morbidity were not available to enable firm statements about most other infectious diseases. Fertility control was satisfactory, with a moderately high couple protection rate, and a relatively stable and low birth rate. However, non-terminal methods of birth control were not used. Effective referral care had been established at a cost the community could afford. Data collection was accurate, with most events under scrutiny being captured. However, retrieval of past records posed problems due to unsatisfactory cataloguing and storage.

Vital statistics from 1982 to 1989

	Baseline 1982–84	Present status 1987–1989		HFA targets 1990
		SEWA Rural	Government Gujarat/India	
Crude birth rate (CBR)/1000 population	35.6	27.0	29.6	27.0
Maternal mortality ratio/ 100 000 live births	3.1	5.0	5.0	2.3
Infant mortality rate/1000 live births	172.0	89.2	104.0	87
Couple protection rate (%)	36.9	61.8	42.7	42

Over the years, there has been an increase in the general level of health awareness in the community. Some programmes for socioeconomic upliftment have been launched and efforts in environmental sanitation have been initiated. However, community participation in most health programmes is at best modest, and self-reliance of the community remains elusive.

SEWA Rural experience has been an almost lone success story among a series of NGO–GO collaborations that have misfired, especially in the health sector. Undoubtedly, the Government of Gujarat deserves a fair share of credit in making this collaboration a success. However, it is necessary to be careful in drawing generalizations about such collaborative efforts based only on this study and other such experiences should be studied as well.

SEWA Rural feels that it has not been able to concentrate on important areas in health care largely because of having to adjust to the routine demands of the government on less relevant and poorly prioritized issues.

Second evaluation (2003): This review was conducted for the period 1989 to 1999. The technical review team found that the quality and coverage of service utilization had reached high levels and the impact on most mortality rates was considerable. Most of the communicable diseases and epidemics had been fairly well controlled. The prevalence of severe degrees of malnutrition among children had also been substantially reduced (from 16% to 2.5%). There was a higher level of awareness on various aspects of basic health in the community, as seen from the increase in coverage of maternal care (from <25% to >85%) and immunization coverage (from 10% to >95%).

The strong points and characteristics of SEWA Rural were excellent community rapport, project detailing, commitment and empathy of health workers, involvement of village-level workers, meaningful and effective recording and reporting system, etc. All the above became possible through a series of micro-level interventions and innovations. The organization achieved most of the

The strong points and characteristics of SEWA Rural were excellent community rapport, project detailing, commitment and empathy of health workers, involvement of village-level workers, meaningful and effective recording and reporting system

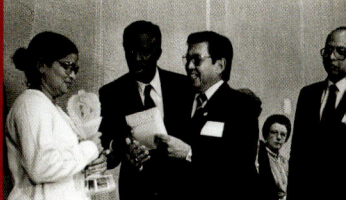

Dr Lata Desai, representative of SEWA, receiving the Sasakawa Health Prize and Statuette from the hands of Dr Suwardjono Surjaningrat, President of the 38th World Health Assembly.

WHO Photo

The achievements in terms of health improvement have been significant and indicate what can be an example for other rural areas towards health delivery

SEWA Rural

(Society for Education, Welfare and Action),

India: 1985 (India)

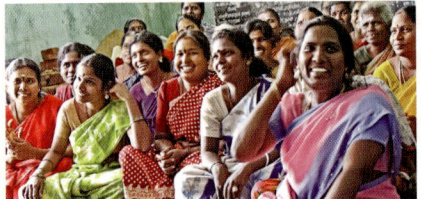 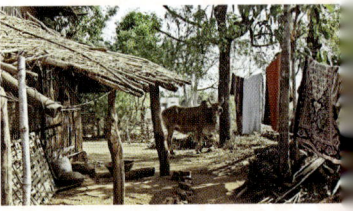

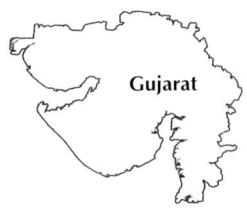
Gujarat

> SEWA Rural experienced several constraints and hurdles while working with the government

targets of HFA by 2000 much earlier, and it has sustained them over a period of time in spite of working within the government system with its attendant constraints. It also introduced several innovations in management as well as service delivery, many of which were subsequently adopted by the government system and by many voluntary organizations. The project also brought out the strengths and weaknesses on both sides, which may be profitably drawn upon if the government wants to involve more voluntary groups and the community in rural health care, particularly in interior areas, where government services are far from satisfactory.

Constraints: SEWA Rural experienced several constraints and hurdles while working with the government. Some of the operational difficulties were satisfactorily resolved over time, while others remained unsettled. These included undue emphasis on achievement of targets, frequent delays in the release of grants and supplies, and interruption in the smooth partnership with the government due to frequent transfers of senior officials. There were a couple of areas where SEWA Rural could not deliver to its own expectations and satisfaction. One of them was the inability to raise comprehensive community participation to its highest level, i.e. involving the community in all stages of planning, implementation, monitoring and reviewing the services and programmes. It was also unable to sustain the village health committees on a long-term basis. SEWA Rural could not do much to effectively address other important public health issues, such as the provision of safe drinking water and sanitation, and combating use of alcohol and tobacco.

Lessons learnt: The rich experience of managing a formal primary health centre by SEWA Rural provides many valuable and far-reaching lessons for different sectors and stakeholders. An important conclusion is that investment in strengthening and empowering the village-based cadre of health volunteers (TBAs, AWWs and MCH workers) is critical for any community-based intervention and in making the services reach every member of the community. It is important to adequately fulfil the community's felt need in making curative care easily available at the village level with proper referral linkages. This would enhance the credibility and acceptance of health workers in promoting other preventive and health education/awareness-building services.

In order to foster an NGO–GO partnership, pragmatic understanding and a sense of appreciation of the strengths and weaknesses of both sides are required. It is imperative to grant some flexibility and relax bureaucratic norms so that distinct NGO characteristics such as innovativeness, creativity and volunteerism are preserved and nourished.

Encouraging fallouts of the NGO–GO partnership experiment: It is encouraging to note that the State Government has shown willingness to introduce some of the effective interventions tried out by SEWA Rural into their larger system. Examples of these are the use of pre-sterilized delivery packs, fixed days for different services, a simplified management information system (MIS) with the subcentre as a unit, involvement of workers in micro-planning and target-setting exercises, strengthening the cadres of grass-roots workers, etc.

The Karnataka Government has successfully experimented with a few NGO–GO partnership models in recent years, based on the experiences of the SEWA Rural model. The Government of Gujarat has also entrusted the responsibility of managing three community health centres and one primary health centre to voluntary organizations.

4.2 Handing back the primary health centre in 2000

In 2000, SEWA Rural handed back the primary health centre to the government. It had hoped that the experiment would be replicated with many organizations getting involved in running government-entrusted PHCs. However, this did not happen. In addition, there were frequent and undue delays in release of grants. Following frequent transfer of senior district officers, SEWA Rural was required to repeatedly brief and explain the features of the programme. Lastly, emphasis on achievement of targets by the year end (31 March) affected SEWA Rural's objectives of long-term planning, effectiveness and achievement.

It is encouraging to note that the State Government has shown willingness to introduce some of the effective interventions tried out by SEWA Rural into their larger system

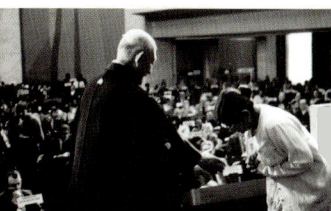

Dr Lata Desai, representative of SEWA, being congratulated by Mr Ryoichi Sasakawa.
WHO Photo

The rich experience of managing a formal primary health centre by SEWA Rural provides many valuable and far-reaching lessons for different sectors and stakeholders

SEWA Rural
(Society for Education, Welfare and Action),
India: 1985 (India)

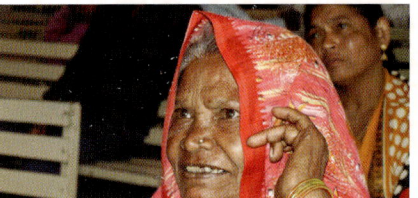 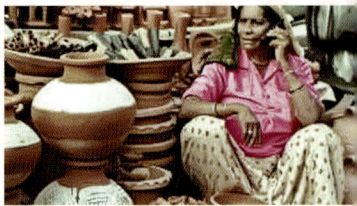

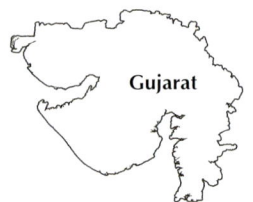
Gujarat

Students from various academic institutions in India and abroad now regularly come to SEWA Rural as part of their field placement, dissertation or project work in the fields of health management, public health

4.3 What next? Safe Motherhood and Newborn Care Project

Since 2003, SEWA Rural is managing a formal "Family-centred Safe Motherhood and Newborn Care Project" in the entire Jhagadia Block covering 168 villages (population 175 000) in partnership with district- and block-level government health departments. The main aim of the project is to develop an evidence-based model to reduce maternal and neonatal mortality and morbidity in resource-poor settings.

4.4 Raining and resource centre for health

Different cadres of health workers from voluntary organizations, government staff and students from various academic institutions in India and abroad have expressed keen interest to visit SEWA Rural and learn from its experiences in community health, comprehensive eye care and rural development. To meet such ever-increasing demands, a formal training centre was established in 1990 at SEWA Rural's main campus in Jhagadia.

Various types of customized courses are offered that are relevant to the needs of the trainees coming from various NGOs as well as the government sector, including those for TBAs, CHVs, AWWs, Accredited Social Health Activists (ASHA), workers for community-based rehabilitation of the blind programme (CBR workers), paramedics in health and eye care, health supervisors, project managers, doctors including ophthalmologists, government health officials and staff of mother NGOs and field NGOs. Students from various academic institutions in India and abroad now regularly come to SEWA Rural as part of their field placement, dissertation or project work in the fields of health management, public health, masters in social work, international development, etc.

4.5 Recognitions and associations

Apart from the Sasakawa award from WHO in 1985, SEWA Rural received the Bajaj Award in 1989 for the best managed rural hospital. It was also selected for an international award in the category of Creative and Effective Institutions: 2007 by the Mac Arthur Foundation (USA) for its pioneering work in saving the lives of mothers and their newborns.

SEWA Rural has been approved by the government as a recognized centre for its various schemes and programmes. SEWA Rural has been selected as Best Practice NGO and Service NGO by the state government.

4.6 Networking and advocacy

SEWA Rural is regularly invited for various meetings, workshops and conferences at the state and national levels to share its learning in ground realities and possible solutions in maternal and newborn care. SEWA Rural has been selected as a member of the District health Society, Bharuch under the Reproductive and Child Health Programme (RCH)-II and National Rural Health Mission (NRHM) for promoting NGO–GO partnership. SEWA Rural also actively partners with other like-minded NGOs in promoting the activities of the Dai Sangathan and Jana Swasthya Abhiyan at the state level.

Over the years, many of its small, micro-level innovations have been upscaled or introduced on a larger scale either by the government or other voluntary organizations.

4.7 Education, economic and empowerment programmes

Vivekananda Gramin Tekniki Kendra (Vocational Training Centre): This vocational centre was started in 1986 for the development and economic betterment of rural tribal youth. Every year, about 100 youth are trained. Thereafter, it is ensured that all the students are placed in jobs in nearby industries and a few are assisted to set up self-employment units to make them self-reliant.

Sharada Mahila Vikas Society: A new organization, Sharada Mahila Vikas Society, was formed in 2003 to facilitate the development, empowerment and well-being of women through their active participation. Awareness generation as well as economic activities are undertaken.

> **SEWA Rural is regularly invited for various meetings, workshops and conferences at the state and national levels to share its learning in ground realities and possible solutions in maternal and newborn care**

> SEWA Rural has been approved by the government as a recognized centre for its various schemes and programmes. It has been selected as Best Practice NGO and Service NGO by the state government

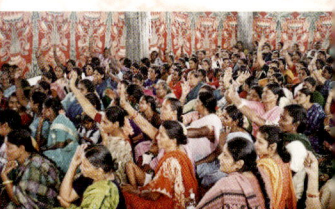

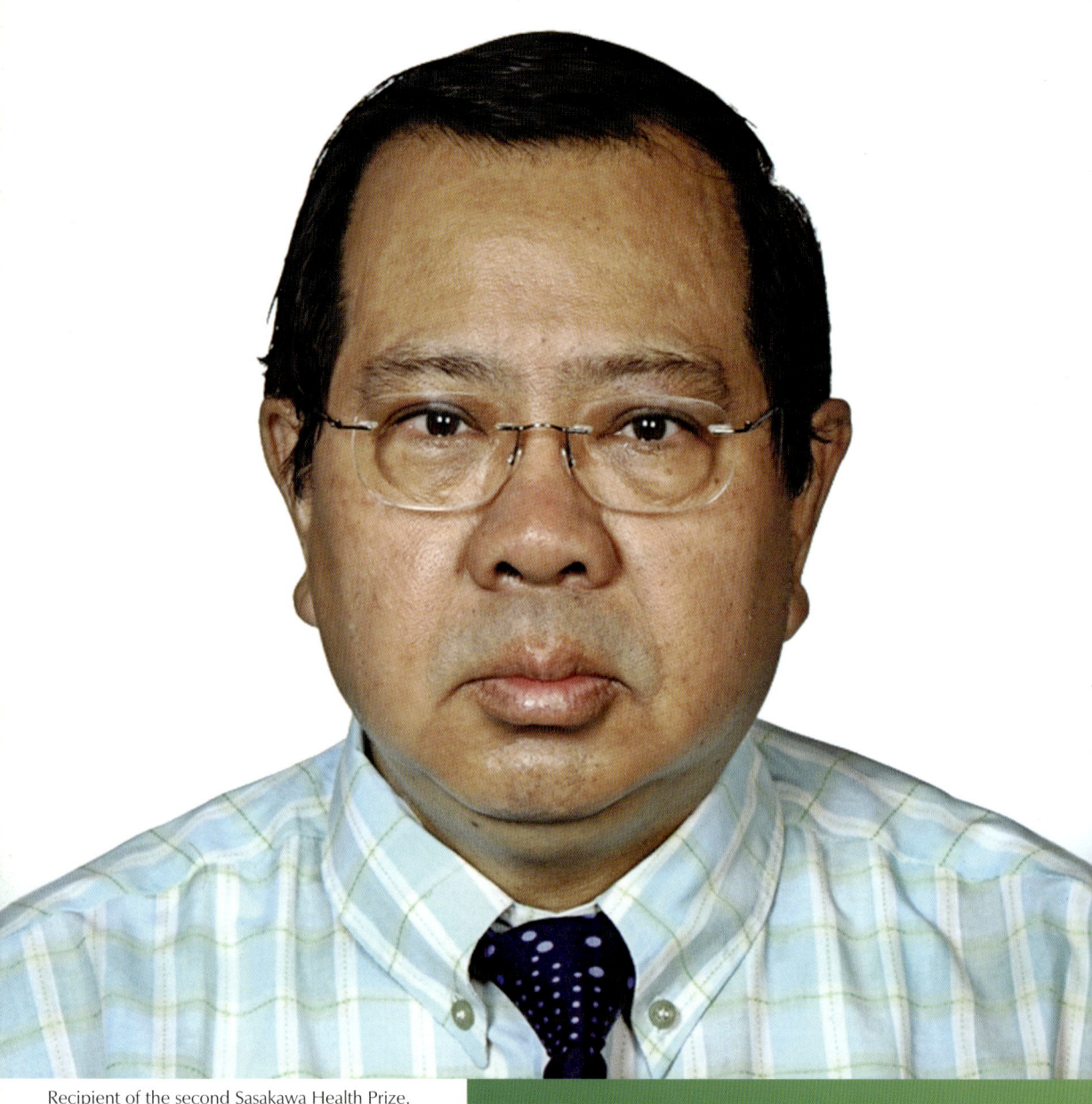

Recipient of the second Sasakawa Health Prize. Dr U Than Sein, representative of the Ayadaw Township People's Health Plan Committee (Myanmar).

WHO Photo

CHAPTER 2

1986

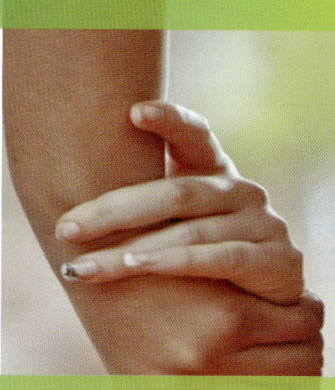

Sustaining health development in Ayadaw (Ayadaw Township People's Health Plan Committee)[*]

Recipient: Ayadaw Township People's Health Plan Committee (Myanmar)

---

[*] Draft prepared by Dr. U Than Sein
Former Director, WHO South-East Asia Region
No.490, 1st Floor, Mahabandoola Road, Between 29 & 30 Street, Pabedan Township, Yangon, Myanmar
The key individuals in Ayadaw who contributed to this project were: Chair of Township Health Committee – U Mya Maung; Township Medical Officers – Dr Daw Khin Htay Pyae and Dr U Maung Maung Win; Township Health Officer – Dr U Win Shein

A yadaw township is famous for its exemplary role in health development in the early 1980s, for which it received the prestigious Sasakawa Health Prize awarded by the World Health Organization in 1986

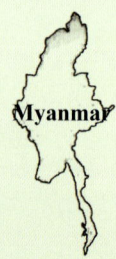

1. Introduction

Ayadaw township of Sagaing Divison is situated in the dry-zone area of central Myanmar in sandy and rocky terrain, about 120 km north-west of Mandalay. Ayadaw township is famous for its exemplary role in health development in the early 1980s, for which it received the prestigious Sasakawa Health Prize awarded by the World Health Organization in 1986.

After nearly three decades, Ayadaw has maintained its high standards both in health and social development. The success and sustainability of health and social development in Ayadaw is largely attributable to following the basic principles of primary health care and Health for All, i.e. social justice, collective leadership, viable community organization and self-reliance; maintaining the balance between local and national priorities, decentralizing planning and management; grasping every opportunity and adapting practices for the benefit of the local community; using appropriate interventions and technology; and having a strong health and other social infrastructure.

The success and sustainability of health and social development in Ayadaw is largely attributable to the basic principles of primary health care and Health for All

The main economy is agriculture-based, with 86% of the land under cultivation. Only 3% of the cultivated land is irrigated and the rest depends on the annual rainfall of 36 inches (with an average of 52 rainy days a year). Table 1 shows the status of Ayadaw Township's health and social development, especially maternal and child health (MCH) care, water supply and sanitation, immunization programmes and access to essential health services.

2. Health development (MDGs 4 and 5)

2.1 Health facilities and human resources for health

Ayadaw has a township hospital that was established in the early 1960s with 16 beds, and upgraded to 25 beds in 2003. The township has five rural health centres and two station health units, each attached to a 16 bed hospital. There are 22 subrural health centres with basic health staff such as midwives and public health supervisors (grade II). An MCH centre attached with a town health unit has been established at Ayadaw town. The Ayadaw township branch of the Myanmar Maternal and Child Welfare Association (MMCWA) supports the functioning of this MCH centre. There is also a traditional medicine clinic at the township hospital to provide health care using traditional medicines and according to traditional practices. The number, types and staff strength of all basic health-care facilities in Ayadaw have not changed much during the past three decades. A few private allopathic medical clinics including one cooperative medical clinic have been functioning since 1984.

Table 1: Progress of health development in Ayadaw, 1973–2008

Indicators	Ayadaw					National* 2007
	1973	1978	1985	1996	2008	
Infant mortality rate per 1000 live births (MDG 4)	63.1	52.8	50.1	35	15.1	79.0
Maternal mortality ratio per 100 000 live births (MDG 5)	70	70	60	60	60	380
% of population with access to safe water supply (MDG 7)	1.0	1.0	97.0	100.0	100.0	80.0
% of population with access to safe sanitation facilities (MDG 7)	1.0	1.0	90.0	90.0	90.0	81.0
% of villages with primary health-care workers (volunteers)	15.0	-	100.0	-	90.0	-
% of births attended by trained personnel (MDG 5)	35.0	40.0	70.0	80.0	95.0	57.0
% of under-one-year children with full immunization (MDG 4)	0.0	10.0	60.0	95.0	95.0	81.0
Per capita income (US$)	68.0	-	135.0	-	480.0	904.0

Sources: Than Sein, 1985;[2] Thein Swe et al., 1996;[3] Kyaw Shein, 2009;[4] * National data from *World Health Statistics, 2009*[5]

> The number, types and staff strength of all basic health-care facilities in Ayadaw have not changed much during the past three decades

SUSTAINING HEALTH DEVELOPMENT IN AYADAW (AYADAW TOWNSHIP PEOPLE'S HEALTH PLAN COMMITTEE): 1986 (MYANMAR)

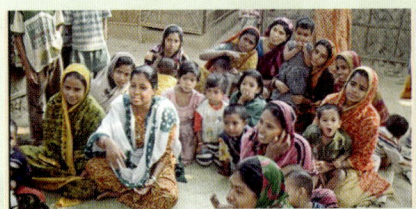
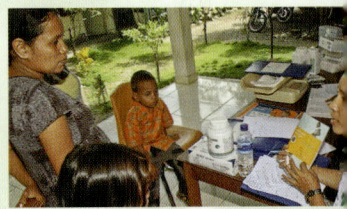

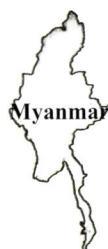

Development of the national health system in Myanmar is an integral part of the national socioeconomic plan and seeks better health care for rural areas

Development of the national health system in Myanmar is an integral part of the national socioeconomic plan and seeks better health care for rural areas, with an emphasis on national needs and priorities through primary health care. The medium-term People's Health Plan (National Health Development Plan) was implemented countrywide in phases starting from 1976–1977, through establishment of People's Health Plan Committees at various levels of administration, from the central down to village levels. These committees were responsible for planning, implementation and evaluation of the national plan in their respective jurisdictions.

The systematic development of health systems based on primary health care and Health for All principles included the following:

- Strengthening and expanding the staff and facilities for providing basic health services, including traditional medicine;

- Increasing the availability of trained volunteer health workers, i.e. community health workers (CHWs), auxiliary midwives (AMWs), and ten-household health workers (THHWs);

- Expanding the range of essential health care to cover all village tracts in all townships, with particular attention to MCH, health promotion and education, nutrition promotion, prevention and control of major endemic and epidemic diseases including malaria and diarrhoeal diseases, and immunization;

- Coordinating development work at different levels of administration under the guidance of People's Health Committees; and,

- Promoting self-reliance within the community and expanding basic health infrastructure and other support systems.

After the People's Health Plan was launched in 1979 in Ayadaw, the township had a large number of health volunteers – CHWs, AMWs, and THHWs (see Table 2).

Sasakawa Health Prize:
STORIES FROM SOUTH-EAST ASIA

Table 2: Volunteer health workers in Ayadaw, 1979–2008

Types of health volunteers	1979	1986	1996	2008
Community health worker (CHW)	25	146	146	132
Auxiliary midwives (AMW)	15	26	42	66
Ten-household health workers (THHW)		2500	1430	1000

Sources: Kyaw Shein, 2009 and Thein Swe et al., 1996

CHWs are interested and motivated villagers selected from each village and trained for a period. Initially, the training period was three weeks for the first batch in 1979. Later, new batches of CHWs from 1982 onwards have been trained for a full month. After the initial training, CHWs are deployed back to their villages to serve as volunteers. When the programme started, one CHW was deployed for each village tract. After some years, as the number of trained CHWs increased, there was one worker per village. Frequently, the health authorities organized reorientation courses on health, especially on disease surveillance and health promotion.

The main tasks of CHWs are to carry out disease surveillance, provide health education and promotion, help basic health services (BHS) staff in essential health data collection, and provide essential primary health care with the support and under the supervision of BHS staff. CHWs are initially provided with a kit containing materials for first aid and essential medicines, and these are supposed to be replenished by local arrangement.

Local village girls are selected as AMWs, at least one per village/village tract, and provided with training for six months (three months in a hospital setting and three months at village level). These AMWs are deployed to serve as volunteers in their own villages. Some villages have local arrangements to remunerate them in kind through some form of incentives, while a majority of them work as volunteers. Initially, one AMW was deployed for each village tract (1979–1995); by 2008, two AMWs were deployed per village tract.

> The health authorities organize reorientation courses on health, especially on disease surveillance and health promotion

> Local village girls are selected as AMWs, at least one per village/village tract, and are provided training for six months in a hospital and at village level

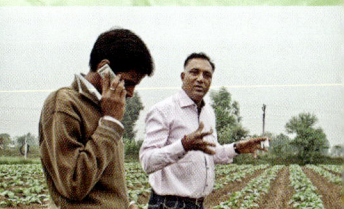

Sustaining health development in Ayadaw (Ayadaw Township People's Health Plan Committee): 1986 (Myanmar)

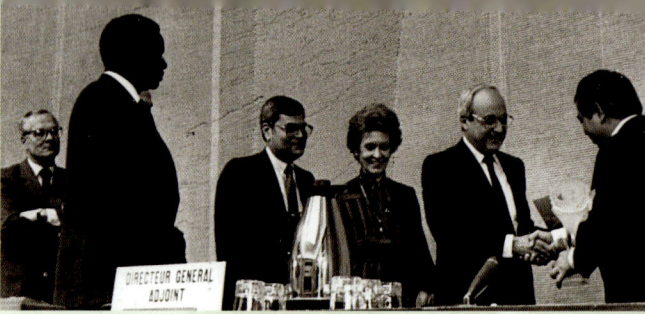

Dr U Than Sein, representative of the Ayadaw Township People's Health Plan Committee, receiving the Sasakawa Health Prize from Dr Zeid Hamzeh, President of the 39th World Health Assembly.
WHO Photo

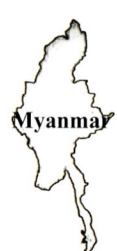

With introduction of sanitation campaigns and a good disease surveillance system, outbreaks of diseases have been easily identified and controlled

The main work of an AMW is to provide essential health care for pregnant mothers, and to assist in safe deliveries at home. If any high-risk cases of pregnancy are identified, they have to refer them to the nearest health centre and/or hospital. AMWs also assist the BHS staff during immunization or nutrition promotion sessions. Each AMW is provided with a basic midwifery kit and some essential medicines for mothers and infants, which are supposed to be replenished by local arrangement.

The ten-household health workers (THHW) are also volunteers; one person is selected from every ten households to be trained/oriented in basic health care including first aid. The main tasks of the THHWs are to provide first aid, guide families on major health issues, collect essential health information, act as first informers in disease surveillance, and assist families in an emergency, serving as emergency health squads.

In addition to the above three categories of health volunteers, traditional birth attendants (TBAs) and basic care providers for traditional medicine were also brought into the health system as volunteers after a short period of orientation/training. About 186 TBAs and a few hundred basic traditional medicine workers were trained and deployed to work in their own areas. Their numbers have been reduced to a minimum after two decades. Till the early 1990s, community nutrition health workers were also mobilized but their work was also reduced for various reasons.

2.2 Principal epidemic diseases

Plague and cholera are infectious diseases with sporadic outbreaks in confined places. With the introduction of sanitation campaigns and a good disease surveillance system, outbreaks of these diseases as well as other infectious diseases have been easily identified and controlled. The last outbreak of bubonic plague was reported in Ayadaw in February 1999. With extensive education and sanitation measures, including rat control measures, no outbreak of plague in Ayadaw has been reported since then.

Sasakawa Health Prize:
STORIES FROM SOUTH-EAST ASIA

Trachoma and its sequel, trichiasis, were the major causes of blindness in the dry-zone areas of Myanmar. Ayadaw was one of the townships that was highly endemic for trachoma in the 1960s–1970s, and had an active case rate of 690 per 1000 population in 1979. An extensive and vigorous campaign was launched by the National Trachoma Prevention and Control Programme. This included provision of tetracycline eye ointment to all active cases, surgical repair for those with trichiasis, promoting the use of personal face towels and education on personal hygiene, along with provision of safe water. With these measures, the prevalence of active trachoma declined steadily. A routine survey done by the national programme in 2008 in Ayadaw showed that the active trachoma rate had gone down to less than 2 per 1000 population.

Leprosy was hyperendemic in Ayadaw, with an estimated prevalence of 3000 cases in 1973. By 1990, the registered leprosy cases decreased to 1550, all of which were on dapsone monotherapy. The National Programme for Leprosy Control, with multidrug therapy (MDT) for leprosy patients, was extended to Ayadaw in 1991. While the number of cases decreased during the next few years, nearly 100 new cases were still identified annually. In order to identify more new cases including hidden ones, a leprosy elimination campaign was launched as part of the national leprosy programme in 1998. In addition, a national leprosy awareness week was launched in 1999 using the mass media, public education and awareness, and school health education programmes. Accelerated active case-finding by BHS staff and health volunteers was done in 1998–99. About 350 new leprosy cases were found the same year and all of them were put on MDT. Since 2001, the number of new leprosy cases has decreased to around 10–15 a year. Taung-Hmwar village in Ayadaw was famous for its high prevalence of leprosy during the early 1980s due to the presence of one leprosy case in every three households. In a village of less than 100 households, a total of 73 cases were registered in 1985. All leprosy cases were put on MDT in 1991. Despite active case searching, no new leprosy cases have been found in the village since 2005.

Leprosy was hyperendemic in Ayadaw, with an estimated prevalence of 3000 cases in 1973. By 1990, the registered leprosy cases decreased to 1550

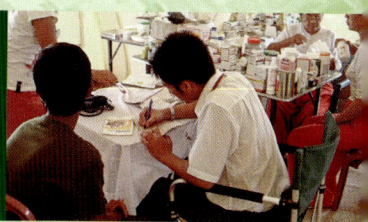

A routine survey done by the national programme in 2008 in Ayadaw showed that the active trachoma rate had gone down to less than 2 per 1000 population

SUSTAINING HEALTH DEVELOPMENT IN AYADAW (AYADAW TOWNSHIP PEOPLE'S HEALTH PLAN COMMITTEE): 1986 (MYANMAR)

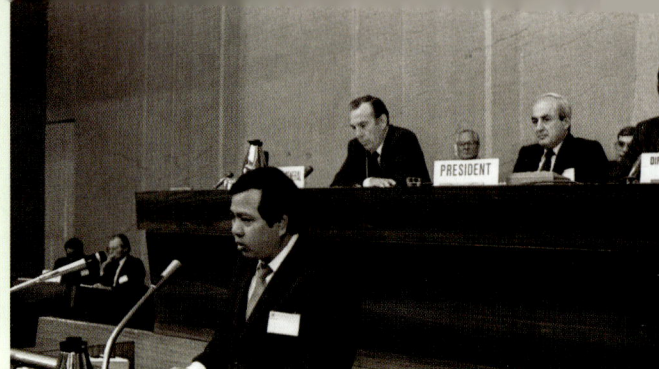

Dr U Than Sein (Myanmar) addressing the 39th WHA on behalf of the Ayadaw Township People's Health Plan Committee, one of the recipients of the second Sasakawa Health Prize.

WHO Photo

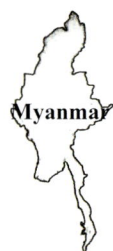

Measles, tetanus, diphtheria, poliomyelitis and whooping cough were major killers or disabling diseases among children before immunization against these diseases was introduced in 1978

Measles, tetanus, diphtheria, poliomyelitis and whooping cough were major killers or disabling diseases among children before immunization against these diseases was introduced in 1978. In the initial stages of the Expanded Programme on Immunization (EPI) launched in 1979 in Ayadaw, the coverage was low, around 60%–70%. With people's participation and the use of health volunteers as campaign workers, a continuous supply of vaccines and an effective cold chain system, the BHS staff was able to organize the EPI to reach a coverage level of over 95% of all eligible children in all the villages. By 1990, with the National Universal Child Immunization (UCI) Programme, the coverage with all vaccines (polio, measles, DPT3 and BCG) was nearly 100%. Vaccination against hepatitis B was introduced as part of the UCI programme in 2005. No poliomyelitis or measles cases have been reported since 1990. Routine immunization coverage under the national UCI Programme has been maintained at above 95% till date.

2.3 Maternal and child health care

Maternal and child health care are part of the essential health-care services provided by BHS staff and health volunteers. In 1979, the attendance by health centre midwives at birth was around 40%, while a very small proportion of births, less than 2%, took place in hospitals. With the introduction of AMWs since 1980, the attendance at delivery by trained personnel in hospitals or at home has improved. The number of hospital deliveries went up to 12% of all births by 2008, while coverage of births attended by midwives at home increased from 40% in 1990 to 70% by 2008. The remaining deliveries were attended by AMWs. This showed the increasing confidence of mothers in trained volunteers, BHS staff and hospitals for antenatal care and delivery. Despite this high coverage of deliveries by trained health personnel, nearly 60 mothers die annually due to pregnancy and childbirth. An intensive verbal autopsy of these maternal deaths will provide an insight as to the causes.

3. Water supply and sanitation (MDG 7)

Water is such a scarce commodity in Ayadaw that safe water supply received a high priority and inhabitants adopted a slogan, "We want water, not gold".[6] Concerted community efforts were made for safe water supply under the policy guidance of the National Safe Water Supply Programme. The safe water supply programme in Ayadaw started in 1974 with three deep tube-wells, pumping stations and storage tanks, and a distribution system for the town water supply. An intensive community effort, with financial and human resources support, was initiated to have one tube-well at least in every village tract. By 1979, the number of tube-wells increased to 63, and by 1985, it reached 141 (with one tube-well for almost every village). Each tube-well was installed with a pumping machine, water storage tank(s), and a distribution system with multiple points.

The entire programme was supported by the Rural Water Supply Unit of the Agricultural Mechanization Department (later named as the Water Resources Utilization Department). After 1990, the programme was managed through the City and Rural Development Agency. A number of artesian wells were also drilled through community initiatives and each well was installed with water storage tanks/ponds and locally produced hand-pumps. By 2008, a total of 987 tube-wells had been installed, of which 217 were artesian wells. The water from these artesian wells was not only used for individual and household consumption, but also for animals and agriculture.

As a consequence of the whole population of Ayadaw having access to an adequate and safe water supply, the average daily consumption of water per capita of nearly 16 litres in 1974 increased to more than 80 litres per capita in 2008. In some villages, safe water reaches almost every household through a piped water distribution system. The time adults spend in fetching and carrying water from a distance is now negligible. The time saved has resulted in an increase in economic activities.

The safe water supply programme in Ayadaw started in 1974 with three deep tube-wells, pumping stations and storage tanks, and a distribution system for the town water supply

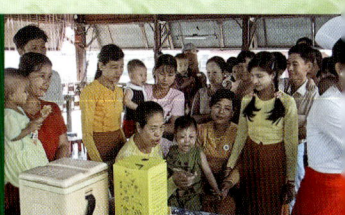

Water is such a scarce commodity in Ayadaw that safe water supply received a high priority and inhabitants adopted a slogan, "We want water, not gold"

Sustaining health development in Ayadaw
(Ayadaw Township People's Health Plan Committee): 1986 (Myanmar)

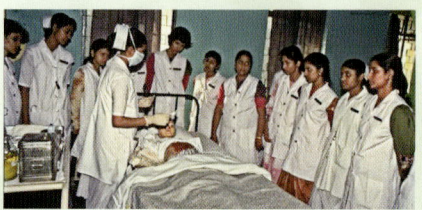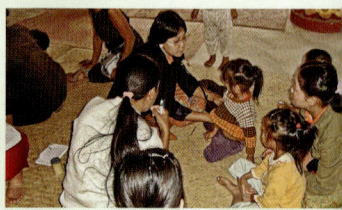

When the National People's Health Plan was implemented in Ayadaw in 1979, there were very few households with sanitary latrines (less than 300 latrines for the entire township). After securing a safe water supply in 63 villages with deep tube-wells, the township sanitation campaign started with the installation of low-cost sanitary pit-latrines. A total of 27 model villages that had a moderate economy and a moderate-sized population were selected initially, with most of them being situated on main access roads. The villagers from these model villages accepted the challenge of constructing latrines for at least 80% of their households.

A health education and health promotion campaign was launched in the model villages. This dealt with infectious diseases caused by unsafe water and human waste, the benefits of a safe water supply, personal hygiene and safe sanitation, and the measures that the villagers could undertake to combat those infectious diseases. Local masons were trained in the construction of sanitary pit-latrines using plastic pans, as well as the production of ferro-cement squatting plates. The pit-latrines initially introduced in Ayadaw were odourless, fly-proof, comfortable, easily accessible (latrines were built in the same compound as the house or a nearby compound), and required a small amount of water. The most important aspect was to provide safety for girls (since they would not need to go out of the village late in the evening or at night). The villagers were involved from planning to evaluation, and various designs of sanitary pit-latrines were constructed using locally available materials. The successes achieved in the model villages were disseminated to neighbouring villages by the village leaders. The prestige of the model villages was enhanced by publicizing the successful implementation. Another factor in the promotion of the sanitation campaign was constructive competition among participating villages by giving prizes for the best villages, based on the criteria of various measures used for safe water supply and sanitation.

By expanding the sanitation campaign to more villages, the whole township became a model for the country by 1985. A total of 23 200 sanitary latrines were built and used, covering 87.5% of the total households in Ayadaw. After 10 years, in 1996, this number fell to 17 600 (65.6%), mainly due to lack of supervision, and inadequate moral and material support. With the introduction of the national campaign of "sanitation week" and education programme in

1996, the latrine construction and rehabilitation programme was revived. By 2008, a total of 27 300 sanitary latrines and 1400 "pucca" latrines with septic tanks were constructed, covering 90% of the population.[3]

4. Education

Literacy is a foundation for universal life-skills. As a tool, literacy has the potential to meet the vital needs of the people, and to stimulate social, cultural, political and economic participation, especially for disadvantaged and underprivileged groups. Literacy skills are fundamental to informed decision-making, personal empowerment, as well as active and passive participation in the local and global social community. The benefits of literacy are transferable, and can thus empower an individual and families. An empowered individual or family would have a greater and more positive impact on the community.

Helping individuals to become literate, in turn, creates positive changes for the community and society. Unprejudiced literacy programmes can empower the individual, help assuage ethnic disparities, and ultimately facilitate the move towards a more united nation. The empowering role of literacy and a literate society can be best understood by understanding the role of literacy. Literacy can facilitate access to information on scientific and technical development, make it easier to understand and communicate legal information, understand health knowledge and medical instructions, help in enjoying the benefits of having the latest information, and make effective use of the mass media both for those seeking greater access and those with no access.

The people of Ayadaw missed the opportunity of having a good formal education programme due to local insurgency till 1962. In those days, children in Ayadaw villages were sent to their local monasteries for basic education, and only a few were sent for middle and high school education in nearby townships. There was only one middle school in Ayadaw town. After the national literacy campaign was launched in 1973, the people realized the value of a formal education system. Community funds were raised to open many primary and

The villagers were involved from planning to evaluation, and various designs of sanitary pit-latrines were constructed using locally available materials

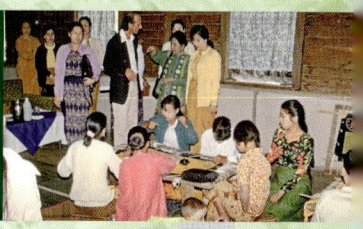

The benefits of literacy are transferable, and can thus empower an individual and families. An empowered individual or family would have a greater and more positive impact on the community

Sustaining health development in Ayadaw (Ayadaw Township People's Health Plan Committee): 1986 (Myanmar)

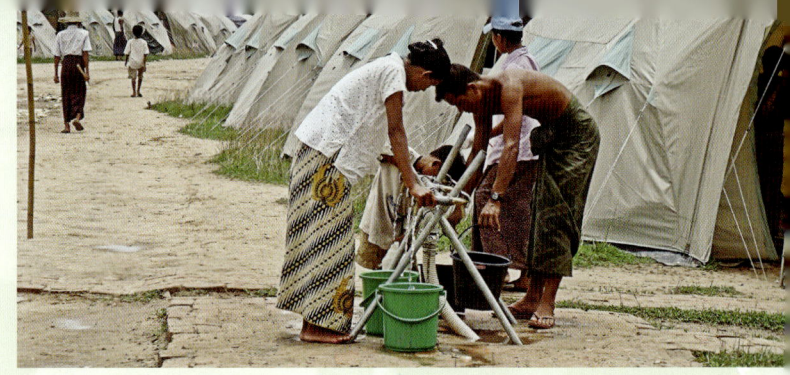

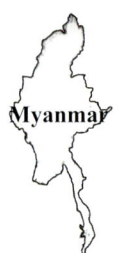

Domestic industries such as cotton-weaving looms, tailoring and sewing machines, rice mills, oil mills, noodle factory, ice factory and seed grinding machines, etc. have expanded in the past two decades. Livestock breeding has also improved

middle schools. By 1974, there were 44 primary schools, three middle schools and one high school. By 1984, the number of primary, middle and high schools increased to 81, 24 and five, respectively, with nearly 20 000 students enrolled. By 2008, Ayadaw had 118 primary schools (three schools per each village tract), 17 middle schools and nine high schools. Modern communication systems (such as radio, cassette players, video-house, television, journals and newspapers) have reached many villages and, with the increasing availability of electricity, local people are now accessing the latest media and news through television and video-plays, newspapers and journals.

5. Economy

Ayadaw has traditionally been an agriculture-based township, well known for its cotton produce. With the introduction of a high-yield cultivation programme in 1981, the output per acre of cotton increased from 250 kg in 1983 to 720 kg in 2008. The government agencies for agriculture and livestock (see Table 3) have supported villagers to sow cash crops (cotton, wheat, groundnut and vegetables) and introduce multiple crops (pulses and beans) with increased productivity per acre; in some cases, threefold. Domestic industries such as cotton-weaving looms, tailoring and sewing machines, rice mills, oil mills, noodle factory, ice factory and seed grinding machines, etc. have expanded in the past two decades. Livestock breeding also improved (Table 3).

Table 3: Livestock breeding in Ayadaw, 1973–74 to 2008

Sr. No.	Livestock	1973–74	1983–84	1996	2008
1.	Cattle	48 900	66 000	111 000	79 000
2.	Pigs	2 300	5 400	8 000	20 000
3.	Goat/Sheep	14 000	25 000	30 000	43 000
4.	Chicken	14 000	69 000	150 000	16 000

Sources: Thein Swe et al., 1996; Kyaw Shein, 2009

Two major cash crops were introduced in the past four decades in Ayadaw. One is called *thannakha*. It is a tropical forest tree grown in the dry-zone area of Myanmar, whose bark and trunk are used to make a paste that is used as a cosmetic by ladies. Myanmar *thannakha* is famous for its oil-absorbing capacity, good scent, and protection against sunburn. Myanmar ladies are famous for the colour and quality of their skin due to the regular use of *thannakha* since childhood. The demand for *thannakha* led to heavy cutting of *thannakha* trees from the natural forest. The natural trees were almost depleted and became a rarity. In the 1980s, many *thannakha* trees were planted as part of household gardening and people started earning by cutting and selling the tree trunks only. The tree regrew and was sold again every five years. A one foot, 20-inch diameter *thannakha* tree trunk costs around US$ 10/- in the retail market. An acre with 12 000 *thannakha* trees could provide an income of nearly Myanmar Kyat 17 million (approximately US$ 170 000/-) every five years.

Another crop is the betel vine leaf (*Piper betle*), of which there are large plantations of several acres. The Myanmar version of *paan* or betel quid (called *kun-ya*) is chewed to freshen the breath, cleanse the mouth and for digestive purposes. It is prepared with different flavours and contents, but normally contains the basic materials, i.e. betel vine leaf, combined with areca nut (betel nut) and slaked lime paste. Chewing betel quid (*kun-ya*) is deeply rooted in the traditional culture of Myanmar, as in all South- and South-East Asian nations. The Myanmar people argue that *kun* or *kun-ya* (betel nut and betel vine leaf), *hsey* (tobacco – cigarettes/cheroots) and *laphet* (fermented tea-leaves) are the three essential delicacies which should be served to guests at home, weddings and at other ceremonies. People feel that it would be impolite to refuse a betel quid or cigarette/cheroot, when someone offers it as a token of friendship and hospitality, particularly in rural areas. People attending marriage receptions or ordination ceremonies are usually offered betel quid, a cigarette or cheroot as a gesture of welcome.

Chewing betel leaf with areca nut and tobacco (betel quid) is a major cause of oral and laryngeal cancer. Despite education campaigns and prohibiting *paan*-spitting in public places, chewing betel quid by males and females (especially those between 10 and 30 years of age) has increased in Myanmar in recent years. The increasing number of people chewing betel and tobacco can be noted from the mushrooming of betel quid (*kun-ya*) kiosks in every street corner, both in rural and urban areas.

Sasakawa Health Prize:
STORIES FROM SOUTH-EAST ASIA

Myanmar *thannakha* is famous for its oil-absorbing capacity, good scent, and protection against sunburn

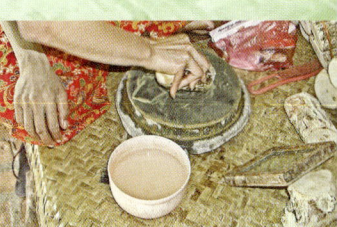

With the introduction of a high-yield cultivation programme in 1981, the output per acre of cotton increased from 250 kg in 1983 to 720 kg in 2008

Sustaining health development in Ayadaw (Ayadaw Township People's Health Plan Committee): 1986 (Myanmar)

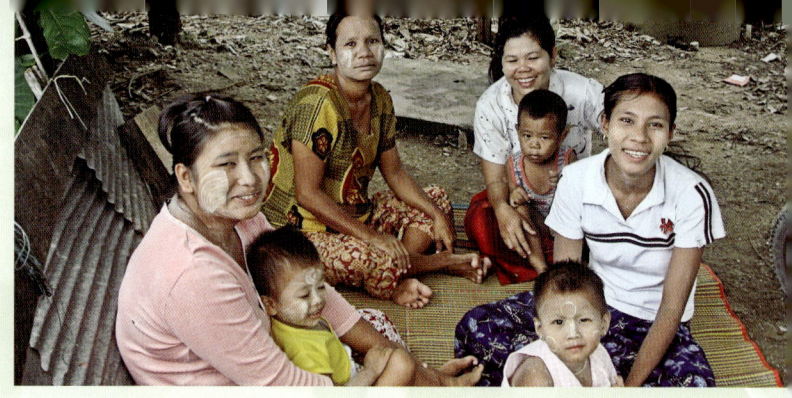

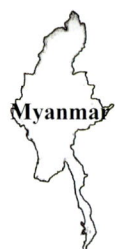

Chewing betel leaf with areca nut and tobacco (betel quid) is a major cause of oral and laryngeal cancer

After obtaining surplus water from artesian and deep tube-wells, the people of Ayadaw started planting betel vines. Ayadaw has over 1000 acres of betel vine plantations with an annual production of 12.5 million kg. This has created an additional regular income for the people, but they have to be aware of the danger of chewing betel quid.

Another "first" for Ayadaw was the use of alternative fuel in lieu of forest firewood. Ayadaw has a small forest area, and most of the dried and cut branches of trees including dried leaves were used as fuel. After demonstrations that alternative charcoal made out of wheat and rice husk and other waste-burning materials was the best alternative fuel source for household use, Ayadaw was the first township in Sagaing Division where all villages immediately adopted the use of such an alternative fuel in 1992.

In 1979, a 27-mile tar road connecting Ayadaw with the district town of Monywa was built. Till 1985, it was the only motorable road in Ayadaw. In 1996, the road was extended to the east to connect with Shwebo, another neighbouring district town. All villages are connected with Ayadaw town by all-weather gravel roads. Now, cargo trucks, passenger buses, jeeps, trollergies (tractor-trolleys), and motorcycles have become the main modes of transport. The number of motor vehicles increased to 94 and trollergies to 360 by 2008.

Till 1986, there was one telephone exchange with about 50 landline connections mainly for government offices. This exchange will be upgraded in 2011 to a digital exchange with many landline connections, even to neighbouring villages. Each village track is connected with magnetophones and modern satellite phones.

With the construction of a township electrical power station with a capacity of 1585 KVA in 1991, and connecting a few villages with electrical lines, Ayadaw's water supply systems have been revived. In some villages, water supply pumping stations had been idle for some years due to shortage of fuel. With the improved availability of electricity, these pumping stations are back to normal. In 12 villages, electricity generation with biogas was initiated with a total power output of 270 KVA. In 28 villages, the villagers themselves collectively established local generators for their own consumption. The total annual power production in Ayadaw is now around 2.5 megawatts.

6. Financing

Community self-reliance and self-determination are the main pillars of Ayadaw's development. The long tradition among Myanmar people of *say-ta-na* (deeds of the heart and soul without any remuneration) and a strong spirit of community self-reliance provided the right impetus for continuous social and health development in Ayadaw for nearly four decades.

Improvement in health status as well as in the economy goes hand-in-hand. Over and above the support given by the government for health development such as drugs and vaccines, drilling rigs, pipes and pumping machines, cement, plastic pans, and training, the community contributes to the main costs of development of health facilities, water supply systems, sanitary latrines, etc. through cash donations and by contributing voluntary labour. The people of Ayadaw raised a total of Kyat 11.5 million (US$ 1.6 million) between 1975 and 1985 for capital expenditures such as building health centres, community health posts, water pump houses and water distribution systems, community latrines, school water supply and sanitation facilities, etc. The recurrent costs for remunerating volunteer health workers and pump operators; for school mid-day meals; replenishing essential medicines and equipment for health workers and facilities; and subsidising fuel for water pumps amounted to Kyat 9 million (US$ 1.3 million) annually. Various financing mechanisms have been established to collect and manage such funds.

> Community self-reliance and self-determination are the main pillars of Ayadaw's development

The community donated the buildings for hospitals, residential quarters for doctors and nurses, and major hospital equipment such as an X-ray machine for the township hospital during 2001–2007 at a cost of Kyat 40.5 million (US$ 40 000). The community also supported the construction of a residential

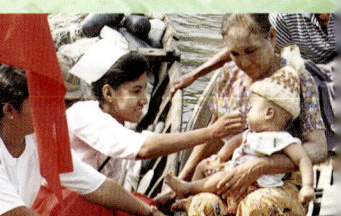

With the construction of a township electrical power station with a capacity of 1585 KVA in 1991, and connecting a few villages with electrical lines, Ayadaw's water supply systems have been revived

Sustaining health development in Ayadaw
(Ayadaw Township People's Health Plan Committee): 1986 (Myanmar)

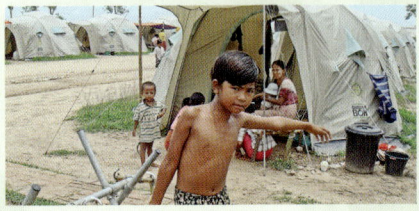 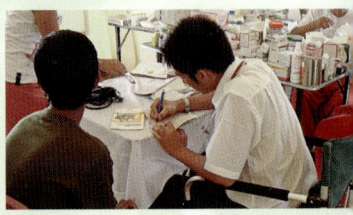

Sectoral professionals work with the villagers by contributing ideas and support for implementation of the common objectives of improving living standards and health

building-cum-clinic for three rural sub-health centres at a cost of Kyat 68 million in 2006. In 2007, it donated the hospital building, residential quarters for doctors and nurses, electricity generator and other electric appliances, furniture, etc. for one station hospital at a cost of Kyat 73 million.

Constructive competition among villages for promotion of water supply and sanitation was introduced in Ayadaw in the 1980s. This process of competition, which sustains outstanding performance in health and social development, has remained active till date, with some modifications. The Sasakawa Health Prize money received by the township was deposited in a bank as a trust fund, supplemented with some donations. The interest earned from this fund was used as prize money for the winners through a prize awarding system. The prize-giving ceremony was held every three to four years. The model village from the southern part of Ayadaw received the first prize for three years, due to the sustained involvement of the community in becoming a healthy village with healthy people and a healthy environment. Outstanding performances of basic health staff and health volunteers were also awarded prizes, which served as incentives.

7. Successive leadership and perseverance of plan

Despite the changes in administration that have taken place since the time of the Socialist Party and People's Council in the 1970s–1980s to the State Peace and Development Council in the 1990s, the health and social development activities at the local level have continued. There is perseverance in adapting and adopting national policies and plans, both in the social and economic sectors. Village-level development depends largely on the ability of the community to plan, implement, supervise and evaluate their own efforts. Sectoral professionals work with the villagers by contributing ideas and support for implementation of the common objectives of improving living standards and health. The focus is on local development, especially in agriculture, education, health, basic needs, and infrastructure.

The collective responsibility for raising funds by the community on a large scale for the construction of tube-wells and pump houses, water storage and distribution systems, buildings for health facilities, health equipment and essential medicines, as well as sustaining the large workforce of health volunteers are endeavours that have continued for almost three decades. This could not have been done as satisfactorily without an effective community organization as seen in Ayadaw. Formation of such community groups in various villages requires representation from the local administration, technical personnel and the support of local leaders and the community themselves, who are ready to assist each other.

8. Sustaining primary health care

In sustaining the primary health care and Health for All principles, the basic health workers and health volunteers need to be continuously reoriented in supervisory skills and community organization. Constant surveillance for infectious diseases, especially preventable diseases, through immunization against tetanus, diphtheria, measles, etc. has to be undertaken since children who miss the immunization in some areas might contract such diseases. Proper epidemiological investigations for sporadic outbreaks of some infectious diseases, such as plague, cholera, dengue, etc. should be undertaken. Verbal autopsy of all maternal deaths during pregnancy and childbirth should be introduced in order to identify the main reasons for such deaths, and to develop an appropriate strategy to further reduce maternal deaths.

Volunteer health workers have been the backbone of health development in Ayadaw, and the national programme needs to be reviewed and revived in order to use them effectively. The staffing pattern and coverage of rural health units have to be reviewed, in order to strengthen their services.

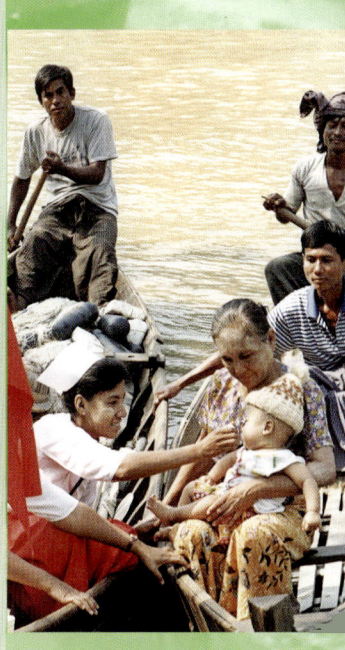

Volunteer health workers have been the backbone of health development in Ayadaw

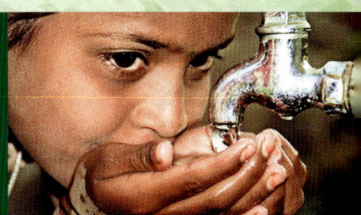

Village-level development depends largely on the ability of the community to plan, implement, supervise and evaluate their own efforts.

Sustaining health development in Ayadaw (Ayadaw Township People's Health Plan Committee): 1986 (Myanmar)

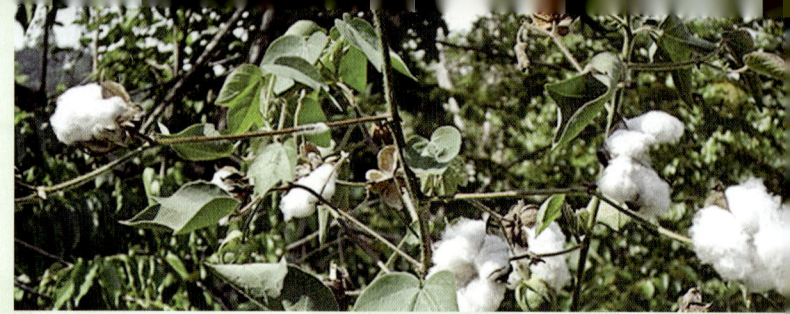

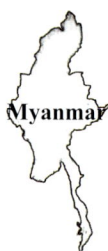

Winning the Sasakawa Health Prize in 1986 made the people of Ayadaw feel justifiably proud

9. Conclusion

Ayadaw is a quietly growing township that was used as a model for health and development in Myanmar during the 1980s. Various indicators and case studies show that, even today, Ayadaw remains a model. The development activities illustrate the importance of viable community organization and collective leadership, having a large proportion of people with high basic literacy, focusing on health, economic and social development, proper planning and management, commitment to change and to further improvement, effective intersectoral collaboration, and joint community actions, which all are keys to success, as well as sustaining the high status of development over the long term. The policy of constructive competition with built-in evaluation is another motivating factor. Winning the Sasakawa Health Prize in 1986 made the people of Ayadaw feel justifiably proud, and the spirit of health and development will remain alive even after another 30 years.

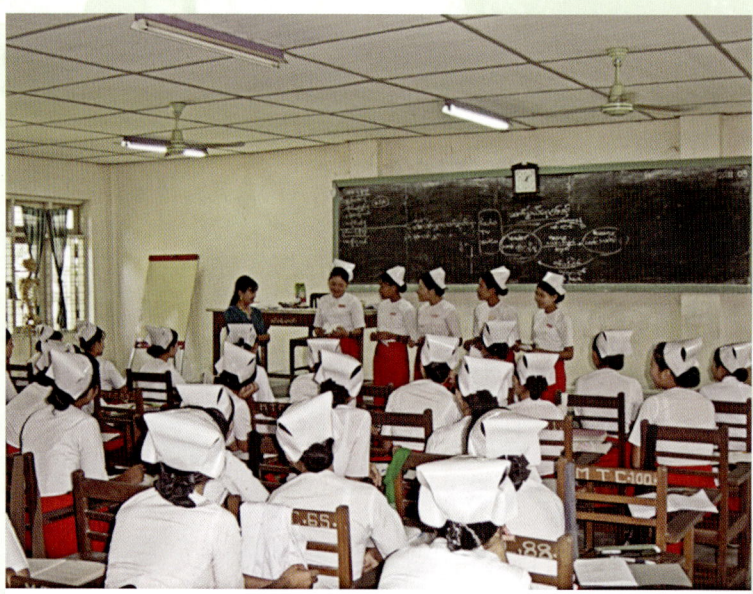

Pre-Services Training of Midwives

10. References

1. World Health Organization. Thirty-ninth World Health Assembly evaluates progress towards health-for-all. WHO Chronicle. 1986; 40: 94.

2. Than Sein. Health and development, a case of Ayadaw. Yangon: Department of Health, Ministry of Health, Myanmar, April 1985. (Background document presented for application of Sasakawa Health Prize to WHO in 1985, unpublished).

3. Thein Swe, Nilar Tin, Pe Thet Htoon. Revisit to Ayadaw township after ten years, 1986–1996. Yangon: Department of Health, Ministry of Health, Myanmar, 1996. (unpublished) .

4. Kyaw Shein. Ayadaw progress report. Yangon: Divisional Health Department, Sagaing Health Division, Ministry of Health, Myanmar, October 2009. (unpublished).

5. World Health Organization. World health statistics 2009. Geneva: WHO, 2009.

6. U Tin U et al. We want water, not gold. World Health Forum. 1988; 9: 519–525.

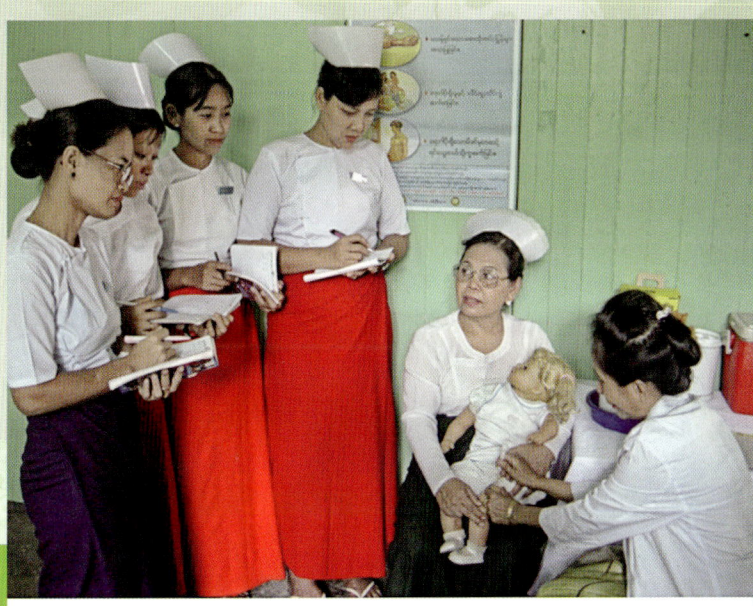

Refresher Training of Midwives

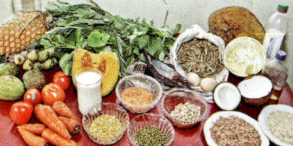

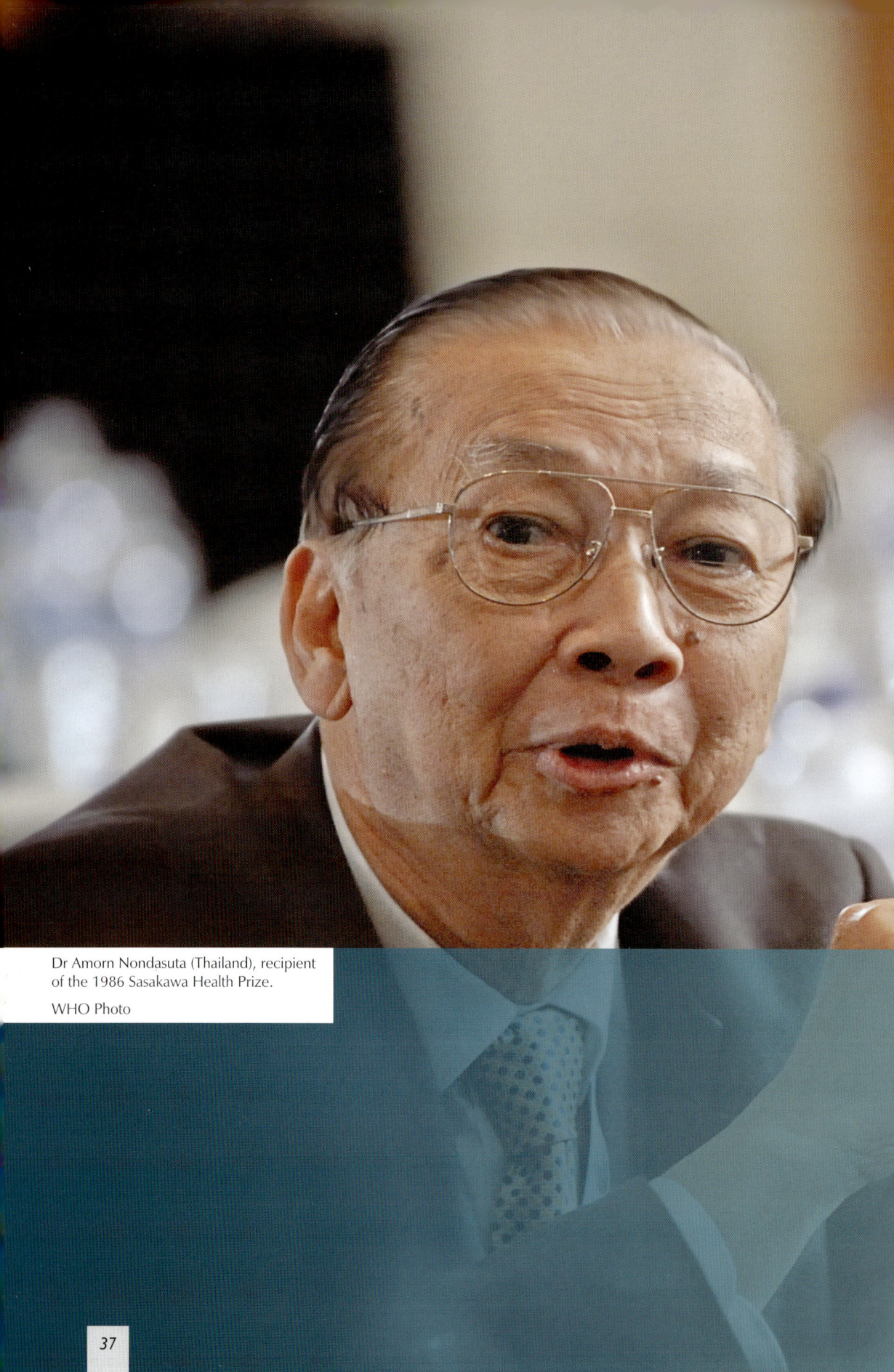

Dr Amorn Nondasuta (Thailand), recipient of the 1986 Sasakawa Health Prize.

WHO Photo

CHAPTER 3

1986

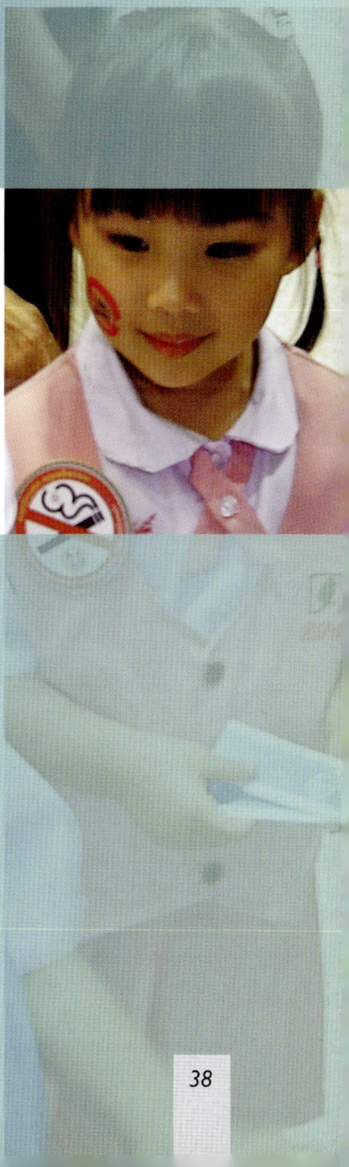

The three eras of primary health care[*]

Recepient:
Dr Amorn Nondasuta
(Thailand)

[*] Draft prepared by Dr Amorn Nondasuta
Former Permanent Secretary of Health, Founder of the Primary Health
Care System and President of Quality of Life Foundation in Thailand

The evolution of primary health care from the beginning up to the present time can be grouped into three eras, each with its own distinctive characteristics

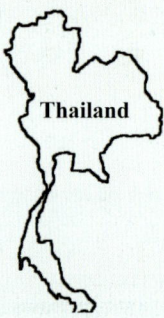

Before the concept of primary health care came into being, health services heavily emphasized the provision of curative medical services

1. Introduction

This article reflects the experiences of Dr Amorn Nondasuta in the development of primary health care in Thailand and in other countries. It is hoped that the article may shed some light on how primary health care could be further developed.

The evolution of primary health care from the beginning up to the present time can be grouped into three eras, each with its own distinctive characteristics.

2. The first era of primary health care

Before the concept of primary health care came into being, health services heavily emphasized the provision of curative medical services. Coverage of the population was a pressing need, especially in rural areas. However, health infrastructure was limited, both in quantity and quality. The immediate concern was how to reach the majority of the people. To increase coverage was the main strategy of health development at that time. The strategy evolved with the mobilization of extra human resources from the community. The first evidence of the community being brought into the picture was the formation of "village health committees". Subsequently, as the situation improved and knowledge and practice developed, the emphasis began to shift. The new focus was on health promotion and disease prevention, which was further expanded to cover management of the environment. Public health interventions began to include high-risk populations as target groups, beginning with mother and child.

The turning point came in 1978 when the World Health Assembly introduced the concept of Health for All and Primary Health Care in the Alma-Ata Declaration. Since then, the community has been the main focus of health development.

Indonesia needed to make health-care services available and accessible to all people. Faced with the problem of a shortage of human resources, the concept of community involvement in health was tried out. Dr Amorn was a part of this avant garde project. The idea was to create health volunteers based on Thai culture, in which care for the sick was generally the responsibility of family elders. Health volunteers were the second community asset after the village health committees, and formed a part of the development strategy. Volunteers were selected from family members using the sociometric technique, and trained in health matters. These volunteers were called "village health volunteers". Practically, the role of village health volunteers was what they had been naturally doing in their daily life, but in a more systematic manner. This design adhered strictly to the prevailing cultural dimensions, which meant that no salary was paid to the volunteers. Instead, other incentives were given such as free medical care for the volunteers and their family members.

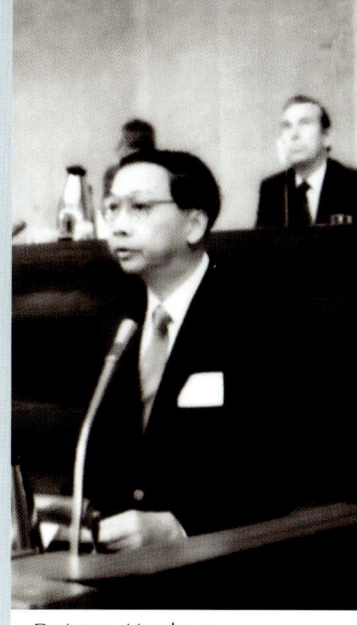

Dr Amorn Nondasuta (Thailand), recipient of the second Sasakawa Health Prize, addressing the 39th World Health Assembly.
WHO Photo

The number of health volunteers has steadily increased and, at present, the total number is approximately 1 million. They have played crucial roles in the prevention and control of disease outbreaks. In fact, since the number of volunteers reached a critical mass, no major epidemic has occurred.

In the quest to develop the concept further, the problem of environmental sanitation was brought up. Again, selected members of the community were trained to produce water-sealed latrines. The idea eventually caught on and a market was created. Water-sealed latrines can be purchased everywhere, even in remote areas.

The other element that was included in the community involvement for health projects was nutrition. This was introduced in the early years. Through the application of primary health care in its work design, mothers were taught to recognize the nutritional problems of their children through regular weighing and charting children's growth. Gradually, with an increase in the number of volunteers and expansion of the community nutrition programme, the prevalence of protein–energy malnutrition has steadily declined and the condition is under control.

The number of health volunteers has steadily increased and, at present, the total number is approximately 1 million

Dr Amorn was a part of this avant garde project. The idea was to create health volunteers based on Thai culture, in which care for the sick was generally the responsibility of family elders

THE THREE ERAS OF PRIMARY HEALTH CARE: 1986 (THAILAND)

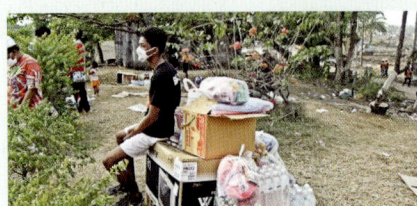
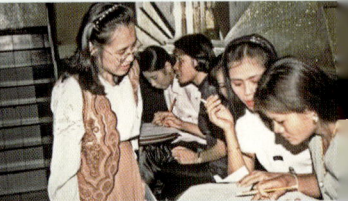

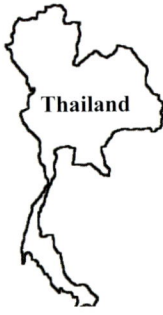
Thailand

The concept has endured the test of time and become the theory that has been applied throughout the subsequent eras of primary health care

The provision of essential drugs was another primary healthcare element that was included in the try-out of the concept of community involvement. Under this programme, community drug funds were established. The aim was not only to make basic essential drugs available, but also to introduce to the community the basics of financial management.

Through these experiences, it could be concluded that there were three elements of the community that had to be developed, i.e. community organization, community human resources as represented by the volunteers, and a good community financing scheme. The stronger the three components, the better the chances of success. The concept has endured the test of time and become the theory that has been applied throughout the subsequent eras of primary health care.

Figure 1: **The three eras of primary healthcare development**

Era 1 — 1978 — Concept *Increased Coverage (CHW)
Era 2 — 1986 — Concept *Integration *Quality of Life (BDN)
Era 3 — 2010 — Concept *Strategy Management (SRM)

3. The second era of primary health care

In 1986, the "Health for All" drive started to fizzle out. Dr Amorn was entrusted with the responsibility of implementing "Health for All", which the government ratified after the Alma-Ata Declaration. To effectively carry the concept forward, the previous operation of community involvement for health was reviewed. One of the problems that stood out was the absence of involvement of other sectors. In order to rally other sectors, the term "quality of life" was introduced, which did not denote any particular sector and would make other sectors feel more comfortable in being associated with the project. To make the term "quality of life" concrete and measurable, it was associated with "basic minimum need".

As with any new concept and idea, initially, the quality of life and basic minimum need (BMN) approach was not appreciated by many individuals and organizations, if not completely rejected, but Dr Amorn and his colleagues decided to proceed with the idea.

The hurdle that needed to be overcome was how to interpret "basic minimum need" in a meaningful way. Brainstorming sessions were organized at the National Socio-economic Board Office, which was the national planning body, to develop a set of "BMN indicators". Sectors other than health were invited to join. This strategic action made the indicators acceptable to most people and the non-health sectors were happy to be involved in implementing the new concept.

After a number of field tests in Nakorn Rajasima province, in which the Deputy-Governor was the key player, the government adopted the BMN indicators as part of the national monitoring instruments to be implemented nationwide (thanks to the strategy of setting up office at the National Planning Board). The BMN indicators have been modified many times and have become the basis for grass-roots-level planning.

The BMN project was introduced to the meeting and a field trip to the project sites was organized for participants to have a real-life experience

3.1 A sojourn into the Eastern Mediterranean Region

A few years later, a WHO Regional Office for South-East Asia/Regional Office for the Eastern Mediterranean (SEARO/EMRO) interregional conference was organized in Nakorn Rajasima province. The BMN project was introduced to the meeting and a field trip to the project sites was organized for participants to have a real-life experience. One of the participants from Jordan became interested in trying out the concept and practice in EMRO. Due to the keen interest and approval of the Regional Director, Dr H.A. Al Gezairy, the first experiment of the BMN concept was tried in the Eastern Mediterranean Region. Since then, BMN has been applied in the Region.

In 1986, the "Health for All" drive started to fizzle out. Dr Amorn was entrusted with the responsibility of implementing "Health for All", which the government ratified after the Alma-Ata Declaration

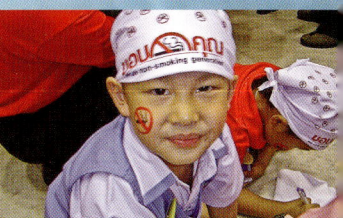

THE THREE ERAS OF PRIMARY HEALTH CARE:
1986 (THAILAND)

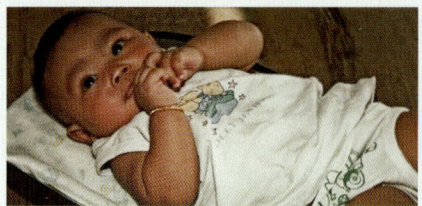 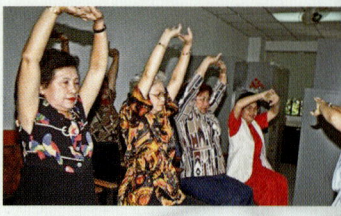

Despite the fact that Dr. Amorn and his colleagues did not have time to work on the organization of the project, it was successfully launched and the people there were happy with the development

To initiate the project, EMRO invited Dr Amorn and his colleagues to be the project's advisers. The first pilot project was implemented in Somalia. Dr Amorn and his colleagues spent a few weeks there to help the country develop a list of BMN indicators, select a pilot area and lay some groundwork on what should be done to get the project going. Despite the fact that they did not have time to work on the organization of the project, it was successfully launched and the people there were happy with the development. The project area was spared from the internal warfare that erupted shortly after Dr Amorn left the country.

The second project was implemented in Jordan. Again, Dr Amorn was invited to give advice on the project. He formed a team with Dr S. Bahous and colleagues from the Queen Noor Foundation. A village by the Dead Sea was chosen to kick off the project. After a short introduction, BMN indicators were developed. This time, Dr Amorn had a chance to introduce the concept of household-cluster representatives as an extension of services in the hope of reaching all households and getting the people involved.

Naturally, when decision-making was entrusted to the villagers, their first priority was their basic needs for livelihood (goat-raising in that case, the same as in Somalia), which was one of the BMN categories. This proved that health must be developed as an integral part of the quality of life, and health alone may not be the first priority of the people. Thus, the involvement of other sectors is crucial to the success of the project.

The BMN approach had been proven worthwhile and survived all criticism. EMRO named the concept "basic development need" (BDN) and the programme became the "community-based initiative" (CBI), both of which have flourished in EMRO Member countries till date.

3.2 Back to Thailand

During the same period, the crucial role was recognized of a good referral system that would link primary care with secondary and tertiary care. The system should not be a stand-alone one, but an integral part of the health-care system. The best way to make a referral system effective was to develop a mechanism to support the system. To this end, a voluntary prepaid health insurance called the "health card programme" was developed and used as a vehicle to refer cases. Eventually, the government took up the idea and institutionalized it into the national health security scheme, now backed by law, which covers more than 95% of the population.

3.3 Lessons learned

The working concepts

The guidelines provided in the Alma-Ata Declaration were not detailed enough to start a programme. The country developed additional working concepts based on the Alma-Ata Declaration. Among them were the following:

1. Simple medical care is deemed a part of the local custom of caring for the sick.

This was the guiding principle in the original design of human resources for primary health care. Primary health care was designed around appropriate treatment of common diseases and injuries. This function was readily accepted by the people since they valued treatment of ailments more than anything else. From that point onward, other functions were added.

2. Function determines human resource characteristics.

In the beginning, there were two types of volunteers, "village health communicators" and "village health volunteers". The former was selected by using a sociometric technique and the village health volunteers were selected from a pool of village health communicators. This method provided a good chance of picking the right person, someone who was socially acceptable and dependable, and would provide voluntary services. However, during subsequent development, all health communicators were converted to health volunteers, and the selection technique was applied to all.

People must be able to design and run their own programmes according to their needs and aspirations.

Simple medical care is deemed a part of the local custom of caring for the sick

Dr Amorn had a chance to introduce the concept of household-cluster representatives as an extension of services in the hope of reaching all households and getting the people involved

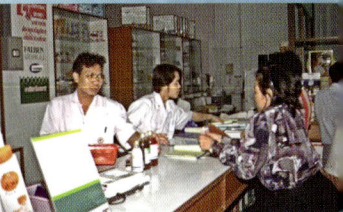

THE THREE ERAS OF PRIMARY HEALTH CARE:
1986 (THAILAND)

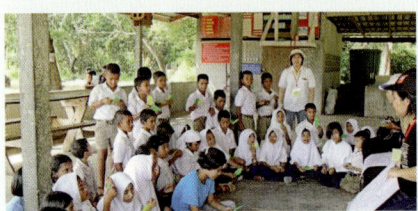
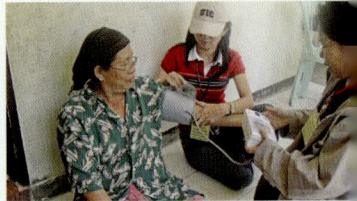

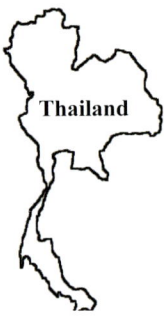
Thailand

The health system was developed around the categories and availability of human resources, the majority of which were doctors, nurses and paramedical personnel

To make health equitable for all, two conditions were indispensable. These were community-owned programmes and projects in health promotion/disease prevention, and changes in individual health behaviour.

Primary health care must be part of a comprehensive development strategy.

Collaboration with other relevant social sectors is essential. However, past experience showed that such collaboration was not easy. A good strategy must be developed to secure collaboration with other sectors. In this connection, the term "quality of life for all" was effectively used to obtain the collaboration of other sectors and the public.

Primary health care needs a paradigm shift of both the health staff and the people.

In the past, development started with creating categories of human resources for health. The health system was developed around the categories and availability of human resources, the majority of which were doctors, nurses and paramedical personnel. Medical and public health technologies were limited to those used by health staff. Consequently, the emphasis of the health system was on building hospitals and health centres. The whole system was service oriented and top–down in design. In such an arrangement, the people were at the receiving end.

With the primary healthcare strategy, the people become the initiators and actors while the health staff assumes a facilitative role. Such a change requires a 180° paradigm shift on both sides, which is challenging. Strong policy support from the top is indispensable.

If the benefits of primary health care are to be appreciated, the size and functions of the programme have to be adequate.

As mentioned, primary health care started off by defining the roles and functions of health volunteers. But if the desired result is to be sustainable, the number of volunteers must be large enough to reach a certain (critical) level of coverage of the population. This is particularly true for the prevention of communicable diseases and transformation of the people's health behaviour.

The primary healthcare system, although an independent entity by design, needs to be integrated in the health service system.

Medical care well illustrates the above statement. Simple treatment may be effective for the majority of illnesses, but more severe cases must receive appropriate health services from health personnel or specialists. Likewise, patients with chronic illnesses should be referred back to the community for continuity of care. Referral schemes must be developed and put in place.

A mechanism must be developed to provide opportunities for people to express their health needs and aspirations.

Such inputs are important for formulating the national health policy and strategy.

3.4 Critical factors for success

The effect of globalization and a shift in health problems from communicable to behaviour-related diseases necessitated new approaches to meet these transitions and challenges: a multidisciplinary approach and social intervention measures. These required a shift in the role of the health volunteer, from one that was solely health-oriented to one that was social development-oriented.

It was observed that the development that took place over the past 30 years underwent continuous changes and adjustments. Everything is dynamic, be it the function of the volunteer, the interest of those involved at all levels, or the intensity of implementation of various components. Ups and downs in the programme are natural and should be expected and understood. Perseverance is the key.

The following factors were found to be critical to the success of the programme:

1. Use the right concept and strategy when developing primary healthcare programmes.

2. Have faith in the capability of the people and believe that change can be brought about.

> **A mechanism must be developed to provide opportunities for people to express their health needs and aspirations**

> The primary healthcare system, although an independent entity by design, needs to be integrated in the health service system

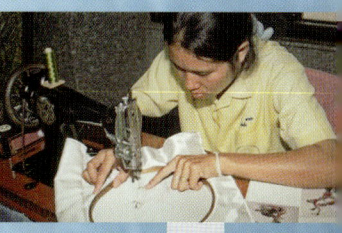

THE THREE ERAS OF PRIMARY HEALTH CARE:
1986 (THAILAND)

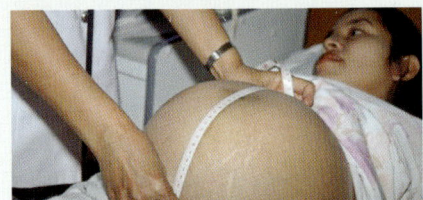
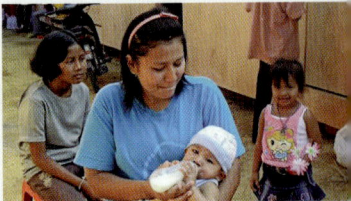

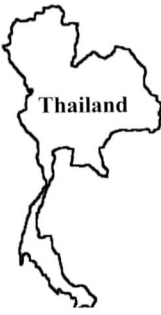
Thailand

Develop mechanisms to provide opportunities for the people to express their health needs and aspirations

3. Put "quality of life for all" ahead of "Health for All".

4. Develop mechanisms to provide opportunities for the people to express their health needs and aspirations.

5. Both parties (people and health staff) should have credibility, respect, trust and confidence in each other, which are the cornerstones of success.

6. A critical ratio of volunteers to people under coverage must be reached (1:100 has been proven to be effective).

7. Strengthen the three pillars of self-reliance of the community: (i) organization, (ii) human resources, and (iii) financing, so that there is a strong community organization, knowledgeable community human resources, and a good community financing scheme. These three factors are interdependent and need to be simultaneously developed. Only through the three strong pillars of self-reliance can one hope for a sustainable behavioural change.

Figure 2: **Era two: integration/quality of life (shift towards development)**

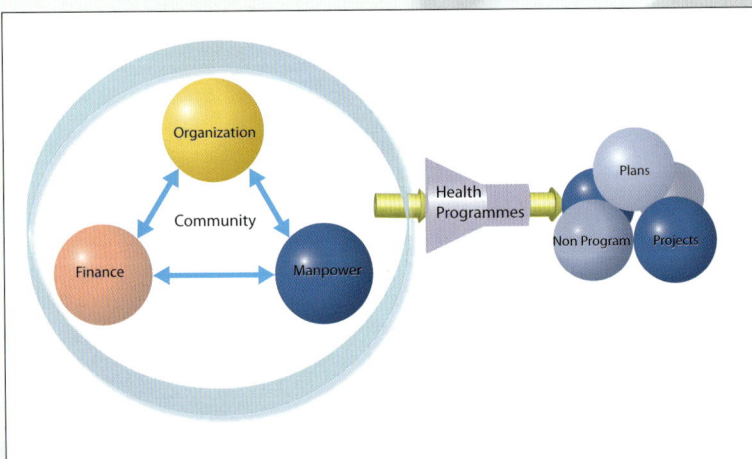

4. The third era of primary health care

There are two possible options for strengthening the district health system: strengthening health service institutions such as the health centre at the district level or strengthening the capacity of the community and people so that they can independently take care of their own health and environment. Going by the meaning of "health system", the latter option is a better choice.

This does not mean that the country must choose one option or the other; it should strike a balance between the two. The decision to balance the improvement of health service institutions and development of the people and community, as well as how this should be done, must be based on evidence.

Such decisions will direct the strategy to be used. If the people's capability is to be developed, the question is, what vision does everyone have? Could this vision be translated into a clear destination that the people themselves accept and take up as their own?

"Destination" is the first major component of the strategy and is crucial to the whole process of development. In public health interventions, the destination or final objective is to eliminate the root causes of the problems in question. For example, what health output or outcome is being envisaged for Millennium Development Goals (MDGs) 4 and 5? The answer is a reduction in the maternal mortality ratio, infant mortality rate, and under-five mortality rate. A simple root-cause analysis of these problems will reveal that the real cause of all health problems is "health behaviour" of the target groups. The final objective is thus to achieve the target group's behavioural change. All activities under this intervention must be geared towards this final objective. Only when this destination is reached can one truly achieve the MDGs. This is in contrast to improvement of the service strategy, which is done mainly by health institutions. This kind of strategy may bring about results in the short term but they will only be temporary.

Obviously, the importance of behavioural change that leads to sustainable health improvement as the final destination should be highlighted. Such behavioural change should be permanent. This requires effective instruments that help people change their health behaviours in a systematic manner. In this context, the "strategic route map" is the instrument of choice because it has been designed and developed to answer most, if not all, of the challenges in implementing primary health-care programmes today.

> "Destination" is the first major component of the strategy and is crucial to the whole process of development

> The decision to balance the improvement of health service institutions and development of the people and community, as well as how this should be done, must be based on evidence

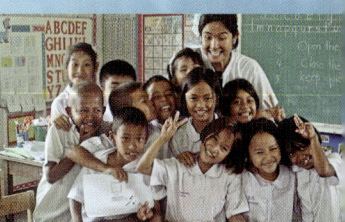

The three eras of primary health care:
1986 (Thailand)

Figure 3: **Mapping destinations**

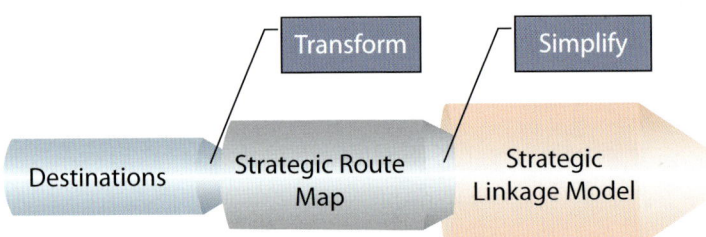

Figure 4: **The strategic linkage model (SLM)**

Components that spell success of a program

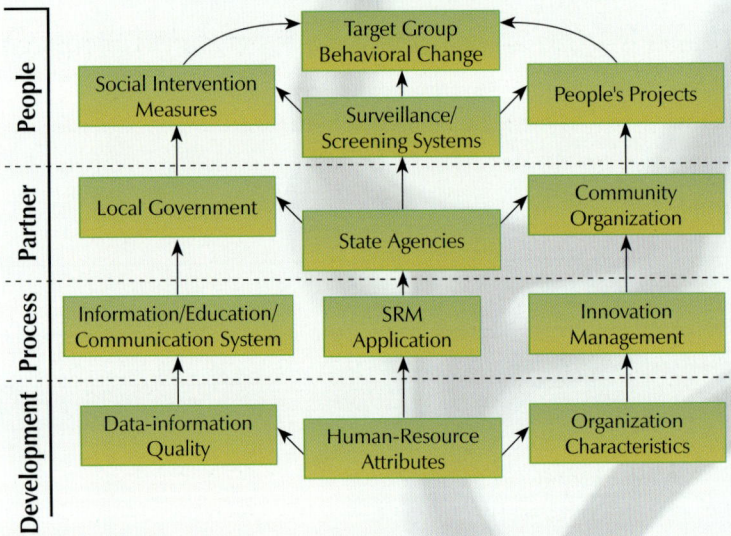

What is needed now is to bring all the diverse aspects of the Health for All strategy into account and bring them in order. In other words, "strategy management" must be used in order to move forward.

In this context, Member countries can get together to develop a destination of WHO-SEAR, which defines clearly the state of development to be reached by the end of the MDGs in 2015. In order to do so, an instrument called the "strategic route map" (SRM) can be applied. One of the benefits of the SRM is that it can expedite the process of development towards a predefined destination and bring about changes in a relatively short period of time. The beauty of the SRM is that the routes towards the destination are clearly defined and the appropriate route can be chosen. Everyone at every level of administration, including the workers and the target population, could agree and set out to reach the destination together, bringing about the elusive synergistic effect that occurs when all stakeholders are striving together to reach the same destination.

5. What should we do now?

In simple terms, the more self-reliant people become, the less the external intervention needed. When all three pillars of self-reliance, i.e. local administration, community human resources (health volunteers and the like) and community funds, are put to work effectively, the stage is set for dramatic changes in the health situation. This is the immediate benefit if a country moves from Era 1 of primary health care development to Era 2.

However, the country should proceed to Era 3 as soon as possible and apply the SRM to make people self-reliant.

Once models are built and certain criteria are met, expansion can take place using the adapted WHO's "Technical cooperation among developing communities" technique, which has been successfully used earlier.

In Thailand, the target set is that by the end of 2010, SRM will be implemented in all administrative divisions of the country. By then, people will assume major responsibility for developing health programmes of their own. It is envisaged that the health scenario will change for the better by a degree that has not been seen before.

> One of the benefits of the SRM is that it can expedite the process of development towards a predefined destination and bring about changes in a relatively short period of time

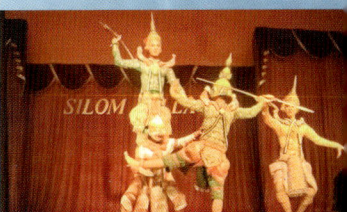

Models are built and certain criteria are met, expansion can take place using the adapted WHO's "Technical cooperation among developing communities" technique

THE THREE ERAS OF PRIMARY HEALTH CARE: 1986 (THAILAND)

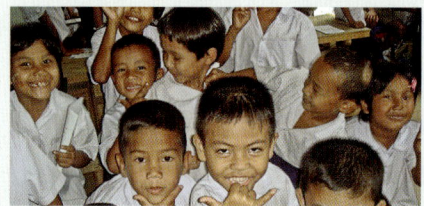
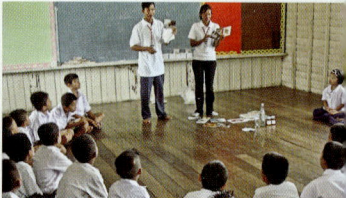

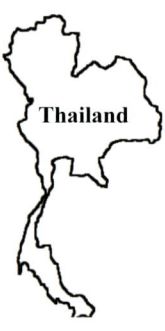

The three pillars of self-reliance could be used as a basis for programme development and are applicable in any country

6. In retrospect

6.1 An analogy of success

The realization of primary health care is analogous to horticultural practice. To produce a good yield, at least three favourable components are needed: good seed, good soil with light and water, and good gardening practices.

Good seed: The concept of BDN/SRM is like a good seed. It needs the right environment in order to sprout. If the environment is not conducive, as is found in some situations, it would not sprout.

Good soil with light and water: The community, i.e. the soil, must be strengthened and empowered. Water, or a financing scheme, must be put in place in order to keep the plant alive. Above all, as light is essential for plants, a policy to empower the people to make decisions must be there.

Good gardening practices: After sprouting, the seedlings must be carefully tended. They must be appropriately fertilized to ensure that the soil would not be damaged, protected from harmful diseases, and guarded against marauding insects. Likewise, people's projects must be supported with the right technology from relevant sectors, and guarded against unfavourable conditions.

The three pillars of self-reliance could be used as a basis for programme development and are applicable in any country.

6.2 Soul-searching

Now that primary health care is being revitalized, thanks to the initiative of the Director-General of WHO, we should see the opportunity to move forward.

6.3 Have faith in people

Let us stop to think whether we believe in the power of our people, especially those at the grass-roots level, to take development into their own hands. This is the most important aspect of all development, including health.

Experience in dealing with primary health care has shown that the challenge that must be dealt with at an early stage is the attitude of the health staff, which may go against this concept. A paradigm shift is necessary before good things happen.

It is time to do some soul-searching. "Do we believe in our people? Are we ready to change our concepts and attitudes?" If the answer is "yes", then we could embark on a road that leads to a totally new destination and primary health care will assume a new look. A whole new world will open up before us. But If the answer is "no", then our programme will assume the same old "service outlook" with no clear-cut destination as to what would happen to the people because they are at the receiving end. This approach taken during the past 30 years has been proved a failure.

We should look at primary health care with a new perspective. We should ask ourselves if we have faith in the people and in what we will do for them. If we do, then we should have the courage to hold on to what we believe in and keep building on innovations. Anything is possible!

7. Epilogue

This document presents the concepts and experiences of Dr Amorn in primary health care during the past 30 years. The main purpose is to put his experiences on record. This is not to propose a ready-made model to be exported "as is" to other countries. The concepts and lessons learned in a country may be valid elsewhere but should be tried, tested and modified according to the country's needs before being widely implemented.

We must believe in the power of our people, especially those at the grass-roots level, to take development into their own hands

> Experience in dealing with primary health care has shown that the challenge that must be dealt with at an early stage is the attitude of the health staff, which may go against this concept

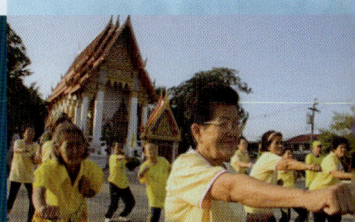

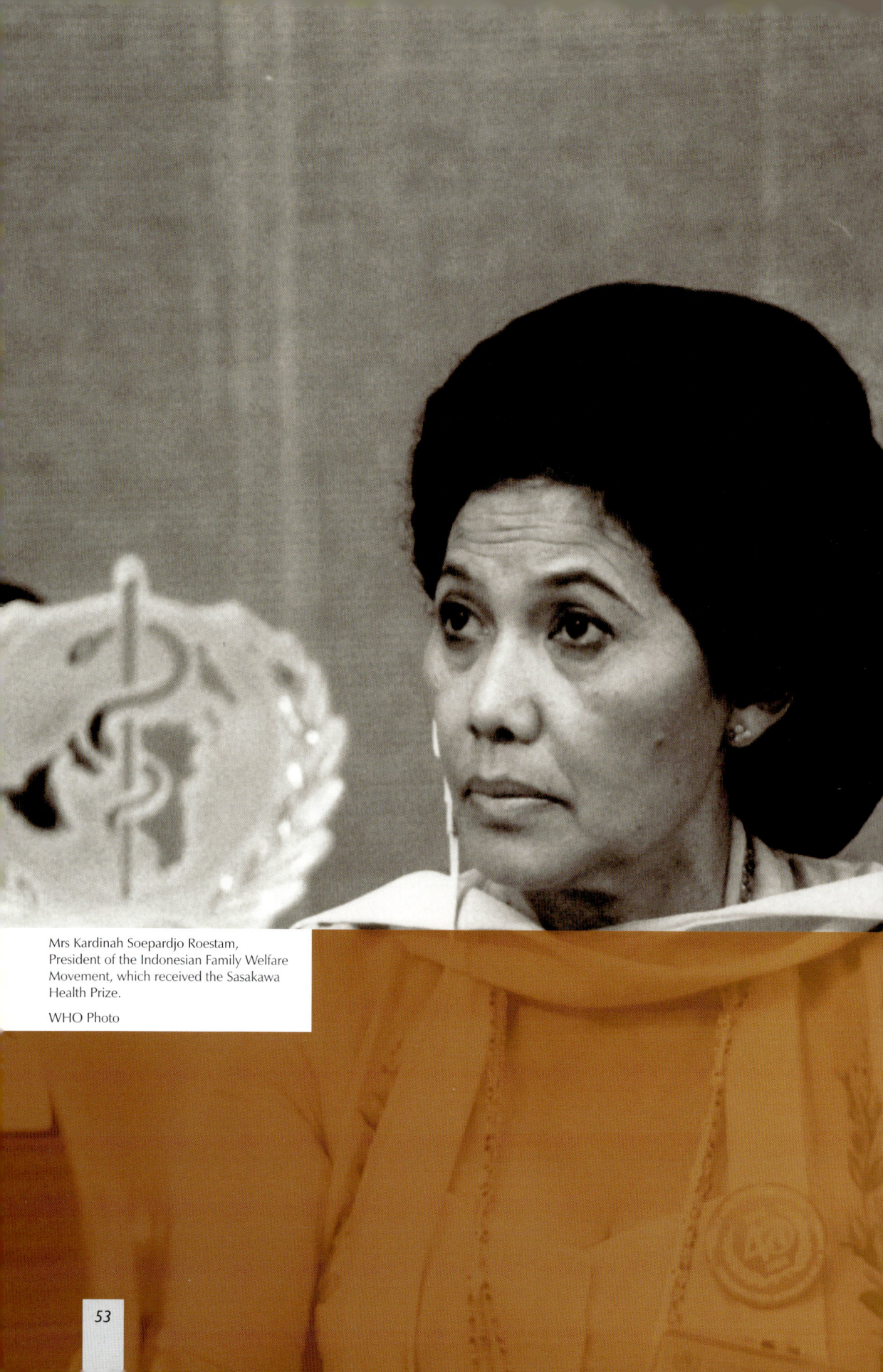

Mrs Kardinah Soepardjo Roestam, President of the Indonesian Family Welfare Movement, which received the Sasakawa Health Prize.

WHO Photo

CHAPTER 4

1988

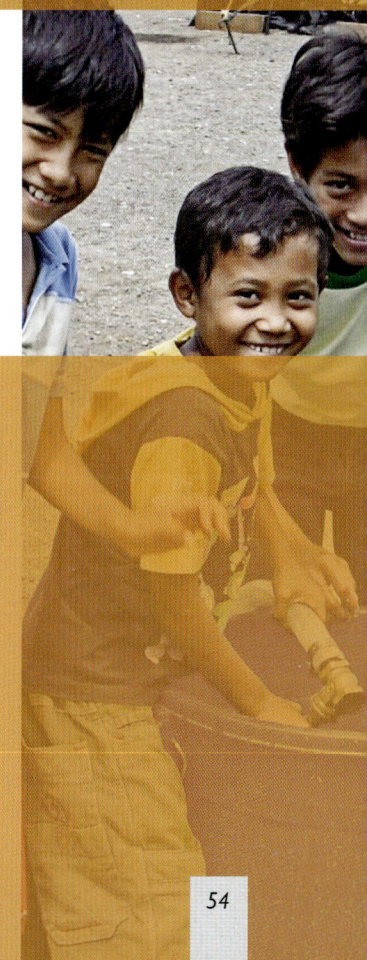

Family Welfare Movement (Pembinaan Kesejahteraan Keluarga - PKK) and its achievements in national development: Indonesia[*]

Recipient: Indonesian Family Welfare Movement (PKK) (Indonesia)

---

[*] Draft prepared by Dr Palitha Abeykoon
Former Director, WHO South-East Asia Region
17, Horton Towers, Colombo 8, Sri Lanka

Women in Indonesia, whether as citizens or human resources for development, have the same rights, obligations and opportunities as men

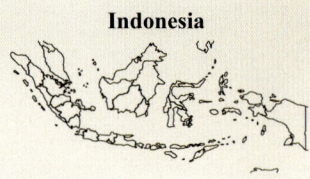

Indonesia

1. Introduction

Women in Indonesia, whether as citizens or human resources for development, have the same rights, obligations and opportunities as men. This equality is obvious in all community activities and development. For these reasons, women's status and participation in the development of the community should be accelerated and guided. Women's participation in development enhances family prosperity. This includes development of the younger generation and youth in achieving their potential as human beings.

Women's participation in development has also been stated clearly in the 1988 national development guidance or Garis-garis Besar Haluan Negara (GBHN). The GBHN mentions the following three major areas for women's participation:

1. To participate actively in all national development according to their capabilities, skills and professions

2. To understand family welfare in order to improve community welfare

3. To build a new generation from conception through adolescence in order to develop a better quality of Indonesian people.

These three major areas of participation are expected of all Indonesian women without exception, be they housewives, career women or professionals. Whatever their position, and whether they live in rural or urban areas, they should execute these three responsibilities for development.

2. The meaning of the Family Welfare Movement (PKK)

The Family Welfare Movement or PKK (Pembinaan Kesejahteraan Keluarga) is a development movement in the community especially for the family in order to ensure family welfare. Although it is a small component in the overall development of Indonesia, if every family looks after its own welfare, prosperous communities can hopefully be achieved.

> **Women's status and participation in the development of the community should be accelerated and guided. Women's participation in development enhances family prosperity**

Sasakawa Health Prize

Family welfare is defined as families that are able to live peacefully in terms of physical, sociological and mental prosperity based on the Pancasila and the principles of the 1945 Constitution. It is also defined as being able to create harmony and balance between physical and mental satisfaction with mutual understanding, responsibility and help.

To achieve physical and mental well-being, the goal of family development includes the following two areas:

1. Mental or spiritual: including the attitude that all human beings are created by God, and as citizens and community members who are useful for development based on the Pancasila principles,

2. Physical or material: consisting of clothes, food, housing, health, income generation, and perpetuation of a better environment through educational improvement and skills development.

PKK is a movement that has universal appeal, and is based on two premises: individuals are family members and everyone seeks well-being. Therefore, everyone is invited to participate in PKK programmes and to obtain advantages from its activities.

Families are the target group of the PKK programme, particularly families which need assistance in personality and knowledge development, those who are illiterate and low-income families, both in rural and urban areas.

2.1 Aims and organization

The general aim of PKK is to improve the family's quality of life by supporting programmes that emphasize the physical and mental well-being of all families. PKK motivates the community to work for its own needs, by motivating and educating people, and by giving guidance and promoting activities.

PKK is a movement, not an organization with paid members and membership contributions. Women volunteers run the PKK programmes and they are the cadres that encourage and show how to improve a family's welfare. When it

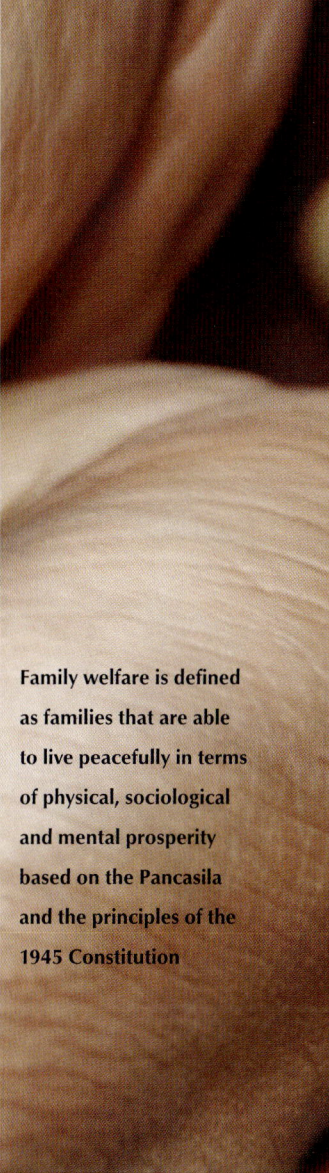

Family welfare is defined as families that are able to live peacefully in terms of physical, sociological and mental prosperity based on the Pancasila and the principles of the 1945 Constitution

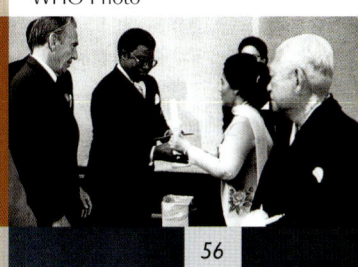

Mrs Kardinah Soepardjo Roestam received the Sasakawa Health Prize on behalf of the Indonesian Family Welfare Movement from Professor D. Ngandu-Kabeya, President of the 41st World Health Assembly.

WHO Photo

> The general aim of PKK is to improve the family's quality of life by supporting programmes that emphasize the physical and mental well-being of all families

Family Welfare Movement (Pembinaan Kesejahteraan Keluarga - PKK) and its achievements in national development: Indonesia

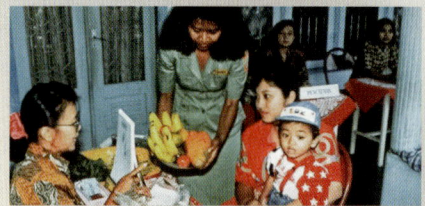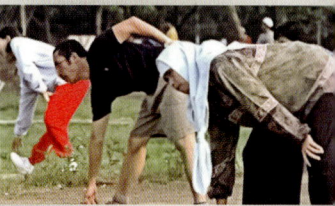

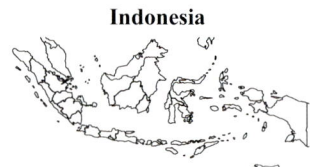
Indonesia

For Indonesians, family is the central social institution, the centre of personal life, not just during childhood but through adult life

was awarded the Sasakawa Prize, the PKK had nearly five million volunteers. Women volunteers act as advisors, facilitators and motivators. The target is women, because PKK recognizes the mother's central role in the family. PKK is a movement that assists communities and the government to develop family welfare. As a movement mentioned in the Guidelines of the National Policy/GBHN, everyone can actively participate in the PKK programme, including men as the heads of households.

The focus of PKK activities is the family. For Indonesians, family is the central social institution, the centre of personal life, not just during childhood but through adult life. Hence, all family members are encouraged to be actively involved in the movement.

In terms of the organization, there are solid organizations from the national level down to the village/subvillage level.

There are two teams that support the PKK: first, the Motivating Team and second, the Advisory or Technical Team.

The Motivating Team consists of women and men who are voluntarily interested in the family welfare of a community, with the exception of one or two paid staff who work full time. This team functions as the motivators, trainers, facilitators, supervisors and coordinators of PKK activities. The team builds bridges between the needs of the community and appropriate technologies introduced by the government or nongovernmental organizations (NGOs). It also tries to be a connector between the local community systems and the national development system. At the national level, the wife of the Minister of Home Affairs serves as the Chairperson, assisted by a Vice-chairperson and several members from various government departments.

At the provincial level, the wife of the Governor serves as the Chairperson and the wife of the head of the district/municipality, subdistrict and village/sub-village level further down. It ultimately ends with the 10–20 Family Group or dasawisma.

The Minister of Home Affairs, the Governor, the Head of the district/municipality, subdistrict and the head of the village/sub-village are the supervisors of the Motivating Teams at the respective administrative levels.

The advisory or technical team comprises representatives of government departments that have programmes to be carried out in the community such as the departments of home affairs, agriculture, education, health, information, social affairs, labour, cooperatives, small industry, religions, and so on. This team is responsible for developing the technical guidance or support for the programmes carried out by the PKK.

3. PKK programmes

PKK has 10 basic programmes which are briefly described below.

1. Comprehensive and practical application of the *Pancasila*

The *Pancasila* or the "five principles" is Indonesia's national ideology. It consists of five inseparable principles drawn from the ancient cultural values of the nation. This programme, therefore, is intended to perpetuate national cultural values and devotion to God in everyday life, to respect human beings and uphold human worth, to give precedence to common national needs over personal interests, to practise cooperation and togetherness of family principles, and to obey the laws and regulations of Indonesia. The practical application of the *Pancasila* is through simulation and games, and quizzes for spontaneous responses.

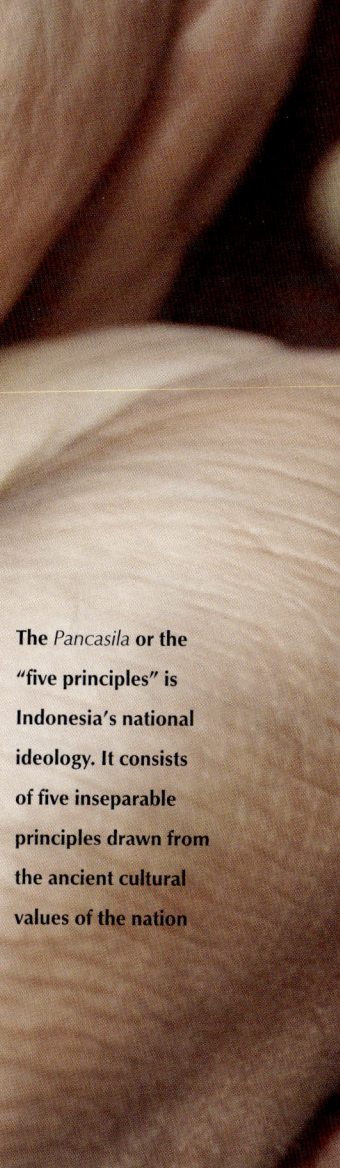

Sasakawa Health Prize:
STORIES FROM SOUTH-EAST ASIA

> The *Pancasila* or the "five principles" is Indonesia's national ideology. It consists of five inseparable principles drawn from the ancient cultural values of the nation

Mrs Kardinah Soepardjo Roestam, President of the Indonesian Family Welfare Movement, winner of the Sasakawa Health Prize, addressing the 41st World Health Assembly on behalf of her organization.

WHO Photo

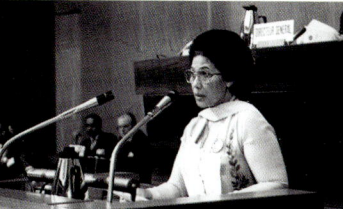

The Motivating Team consists of women and men who are voluntarily interested in the family welfare of a community

Family Welfare Movement (Pembinaan Kesejahteraan Keluarga - PKK) and its achievements in national development: Indonesia

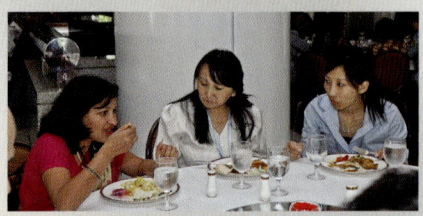
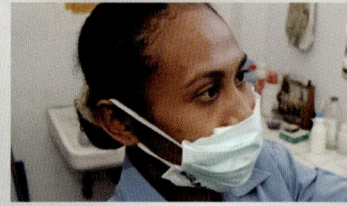

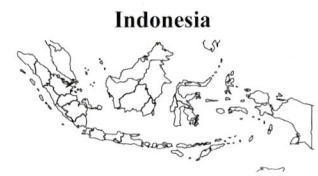
Indonesia

2. Mutual self-help or *gotong-royong*

Gotong means "bearing the weight of something together", while *royong* means sharing the proceeds. This phrase describes an ancient and well-defined system of cooperation and expresses the traditional feeling of familial ties, which is called *kekeluargaan*. *Gotong-royong* is integral to all Indonesian communities, be they traditional, developed or developing.

3. Food

After the poverty-stricken conditions and accompanying ignorance during colonial times, people needed to learn the importance of nutrition for the physical and mental well-being of family members. People should know that healthy and nutritious menus can be cheap and within the reach of all. They should also be aware that many items on these menus are not difficult to cook. Home gardens can be planted with fast-growing vegetables. Fish and small livestock can be kept without detriment to the environment in confined and densely populated areas. Home gardens can also be used to grow traditional herbs for medicines or *jamu*.

People needed to learn the importance of nutrition for the physical and mental well-being of family members

4. Clothing

In the past, poverty resulted in the neglect of clothing. However, today people are aware that clean and suitable clothing is one of the basic needs of human beings. People can easily learn how to make clothing and patch-work bedspreads to meet the needs of the family.

5. Housing and home economics

Homes are the places where families improve the quality of their lives. The first requirement of comfortable housing is hygiene and a pleasant environment. In this case, people need to know how to make a simple, healthy and attractive house at a reasonable cost. People should also understand how to care for it and use the garden or yard effectively. An understanding of home economics is essential for the family's happiness as well as for its economic well-being.

6. Education and craft skills

Since the institution of compulsory education, PKK motivates parents to provide "good" education for both boys and girls between the ages of 6 and 12 years. The PKK programme uses informal rather than formal education. Literacy courses are fundamental for any education programme. In response, a "paket (package) A" has been developed, which consists of a set of literary primers that convey useful basic education. PKK also recognizes the importance of "lifelong education", which of course does not mean merely academic or classroom education.

Craft skills provide a better quality of life at a low cost. Embroidery, making children's toys, knitting, crocheting, dress-making and simple carpentry can increase a family's well-being and income. Programmes such as radio repairing and even beauty care education are given special emphasis by PKK.

7. Health

Good health is an absolute necessity for the well-being of both individuals and families. The significant contribution of good health to well-being needs to be emphasized in communities in which poverty, poor health and ignorance have existed for a long time. Personal hygiene habits and environmental protection are also fostered by PKK. People are shown how to obtain adequate supplies of safe drinking water and how to protect clean environments with proper disposal of household rubbish and waste.

Special attention is given to the health conditions of children under 5 years of age, couples of childbearing age, and pregnant and lactating mothers. In order to reach these groups, PKK has established at least one post in every village for regular meetings once a month. This post is called the *Posyandu*, or Integrated Community Health Services Post. It has five basic services: immunization,

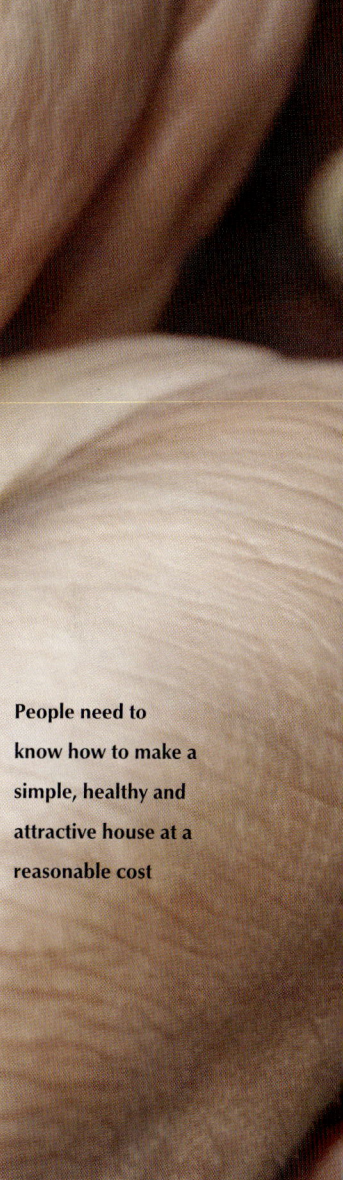

Sasakawa Health Prize:
STORIES FROM SOUTH-EAST ASIA

People need to know how to make a simple, healthy and attractive house at a reasonable cost

Mrs Kardinah Soepardjo Roestam, President of the Indonesian Family Welfare Movement, being congratulated by Mr Ryoichi Sasakawa after the prize giving ceremony of the Sasakawa Health Prize.

WHO Photo

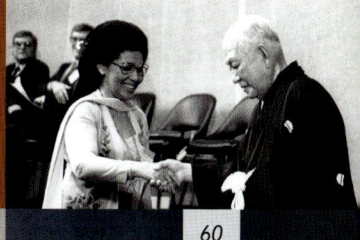

The significant contribution of good health to well-being needs to be emphasized in communities in which poverty, poor health and ignorance have existed for a long time

FAMILY WELFARE MOVEMENT (PEMBINAAN KESEJAHTERAAN KELUARGA - PKK) AND ITS ACHIEVEMENTS IN NATIONAL DEVELOPMENT: INDONESIA

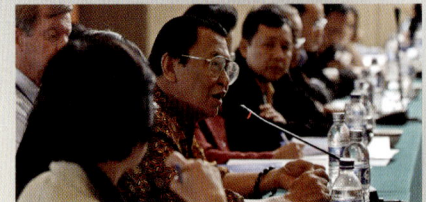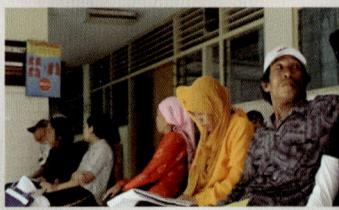

Indonesia

Women volunteers act as advisors, facilitators and motivators

nutrition, family planning, maternal and child health, and diarrhoeal disease control Women bring their under-five children to the post for monthly monitoring of the children's weight and growth, immunization against six major childhood diseases, demonstrations on nutritious feeding, and obtaining oral rehydration solutions for children with diarrhoea. Health education, family planning services and information are also provided for eligible couples. One goal is for women not to deliver a child before they are 20 years old. PKK also promotes small families – two children are enough, spaced at least three years apart. Women are also encouraged to breast-feed their children for its obvious advantages to both children and mothers. Other maternal and child health-related care is also provided in the *Posyandu* such as pregnancy and prenatal care, distribution of vitamin A capsules and ferrous sulphate tablets.

8. Development cooperatives

Cooperatives are a basic part of Indonesia's economic democracy. It is a form of enterprise through which a group of small businessmen can be strongly encouraged. Development of cooperatives provides communities with job opportunities, which are otherwise difficult to create.

9. Protection and conservation of the environment

This programme supports harmony between families, their neighbourhoods and their natural environment. Understanding the importance of conservation can help to reduce environmental damage, for example, from cutting firewood, or polluting rivers due to improper waste disposal.

10. Sound planning

The sound planning of family income and expenditure is very important for a poor family, particularly when there are many people working in a household. Organizing time for work and recreation, and distributing household duties among the different members of a family based on their respective capacities and interests will, hopefully lead to more orderly, effective, efficient and happier lives.

4. Programme implementation

While implementing PKK programmes, not every point of the 10 basic programmes has to be simultaneously carried out. Priorities for programme implementation are determined by villagers based on their most felt needs. PKK activities are divided into four working groups (kelompok kerja or POKJA) and the 10 programmes are divided among these four groups for implementation.

PKK always has a close relationship with the various levels of local government administrators and local departmental services in implementing programmes. In the PKK strategy of reaching as many families as possible, households are organized by PKK into units of ten under the leadership of a chairperson elected among the families in this unit of households. This approach is called the dasawisma approach. The chairperson records and reports the number of pregnant women, number of births, number of infant deaths, number of under-five children immunized, and identifies illiterate members of the families for non-formal education/learning groups and development activities, in which they too are active implementers.

Local PKK motivating teams discuss proposed programmes and projects with groups of villagers. Through these meetings, members of the local community are involved in the planning process. With this involvement, villagers develop their planning abilities and capabilities. Necessary technical information, for example, how much cement will be needed to build a public or family bathing place, a public laundry and a lavatory facility, is provided by various local departmental services at the district level.

PKK activities are funded by the local community and through donations. Government assistance is mainly in the form of materials, facilities and technical guidance. For instance, the Ministry of Health supplies various vaccines for immunization and also provides paramedical personnel for

Priorities for programme implementation are determined by villagers based on their most felt needs

---

PKK activities are funded by the local community and through donations. Government assistance is mainly in the form of materials, facilities and technical guidance

FAMILY WELFARE MOVEMENT (PEMBINAAN KESEJAHTERAAN KELUARGA - PKK) AND ITS ACHIEVEMENTS IN NATIONAL DEVELOPMENT: INDONESIA

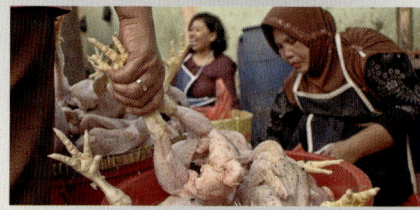 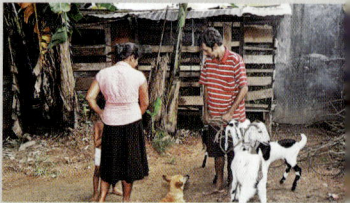

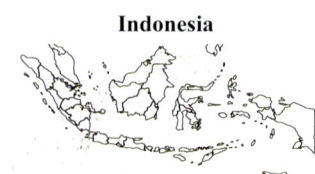

Indonesia

The Ministry of Health supplies various vaccines for immunization and also provides paramedical personnel for administering them

administering them. In mass immunization campaigns conducted by PKK, it prepares the village hall, and the facilities needed for the immunization activity. PKK motivates mothers to bring their children for immunization.

Perhaps a group of women will decide to set aside one spoonful of rice every time they cook. These spoonfuls are accumulated in the households and collected together after a certain length of time. When there is a large enough quantity, it will be sold to provide funds to the PKK. Or perhaps people start a revolving lottery by collecting a small amount of money every month. The accumulated fund is used in turn by every member of the group by casting lots every month. Perhaps someone would buy a pair of breeding rabbits. After they multiply, some are sold and the proceeds used to buy a pair of goats. As time goes on, villagers can own their goats or even buffaloes by this method.

Village roads, housing repairs and construction, digging and lining drainage or sanitary ditches, building public toilets and other similar community developments are carried out by gotong-royong activities. For example, villagers spend a few hours every week to collect stones from rivers, while others lay them on the roads converting them into facilities that improve the quality of lives of the villagers.

5. Achievements

Some of the following data show in simple terms what PKK has achieved. Most of the figures given here are from the 1984–1987 period.

1. Programme for the comprehension and practical application of the national ideology *Pancasila*

This programme is conducted by means of simulations and games. It is a media presentation on how to apply the *Pancasila* in everyday life.

Members of motivation teams who have attended training courses in the propagation of the *Pancasila* have doubled within these three years. The number of simulation groups has increased by over 50% since 1984.

In addition, there are groups set up to help members when there are deaths in a family: 300 000 groups, and rotating lottery (*arisan*) groups to collect funds for community needs: 240 000 groups in 1986–87.

2. Programme for education and training in skills. The numbers who have benefited from these programmes exceeded one million.

3. Programme for food, clothing and shelter (1986/87)

The percentage of village families throughout Indonesia using home yards for growing nutritious food, fruits, vegetables and small livestock was 57%. The number of cottage industries, businesses promoted and supervised by PKK, and the number of healthy houses in the villages increased by almost 300%, touching nearly 11 million units in the four years.

4. Programmes for health, family planning, conservation of the environment and appropriate domestic planning (1986/87)

(a)	Health	
	Number of bath, laundry and lavatory units	673 000
	Number of family lavatories	6 million
	Number of integrated health posts	200 000
	Number of nutrition gardens	1.4 million

(b)	Family planning	
	Number of eligible couples:	roughly 20 million
	Number of acceptors using:	pills 35% intrauterine devices (IUDs) 21% condoms 3% injections 10%

(c)	Conservation of the environment		
	Number of families obtaining clean water supplies:	rain-water	1.5 million
		wells	9.5 million
		springs	5.5 million

Villagers spend a few hours every week to collect stones from rivers, while others lay them on the roads converting them into facilities that improve the quality of lives of the villagers

Sasakawa Health Prize:
STORIES FROM SOUTH-EAST ASIA

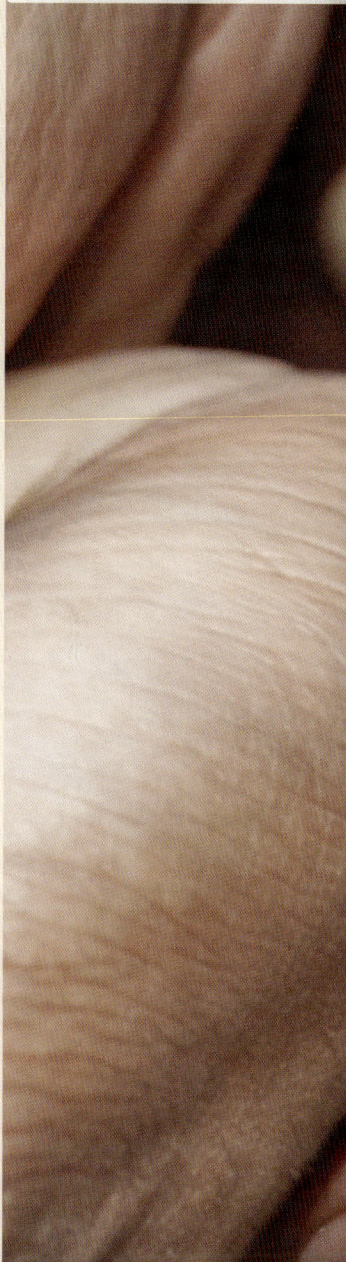

Mr Ryoichi Sasakawa showing the scars of his leprosy vaccination during his address to the special meeting of the 41st World Health Assembly.
WHO Photo

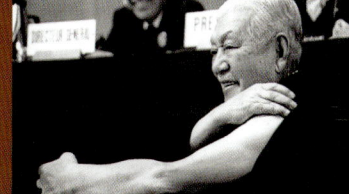

Family Welfare Movement (Pembinaan Kesejahteraan Keluarga - PKK) and its achievements in national development: Indonesia

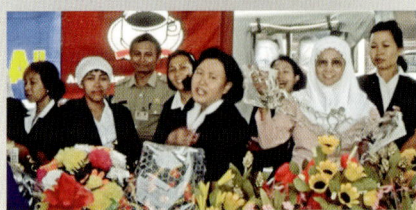
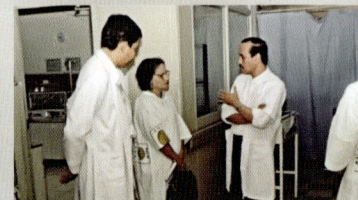

Indonesia

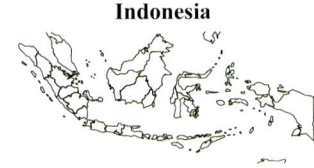

5. Cooperative programmes

PKK set up more than 230 000 small cooperative shops.

6. Savings programmes

   Number of savings accounts opened due to PKK encouragement

   – *Tabanas'* (national savings)   1.75 million

   – *Taska'* (insurance savings)   215 000

   – *Tapelpram* (scouts and students' savings)   611 000

6. Problems and supporting factors

Although PKK has achieved many goals and is widely acknowledged as one of the key movements in rural Indonesia, it faces many challenges such as those listed below.

1. Low level of family education

2. Inadequate incomes of some families

3. Traditional laws that sometimes act as obstacles

4. Insufficient number of skilled personnel

5. Difficulties in communication due to inadequate infrastructure facilities

Sasakawa Health Prize:
STORIES FROM SOUTH-EAST ASIA

6. Geographical inaccessibility

7. Instability of some PKK structures and mechanisms

8. Lack of integration in sectoral policies and rigid bureaucracies

9. Shortage of time among PKK volunteers.

There are, however, a number of opportunities that support PKK:

1. Gotong-Royong or mutual help. Without this ethic, most PKK programmes could not be implemented quickly, if at all

2. The religious attitude of Indonesian communities

3. Following the advice of the leaders as well as their examples is a habit inherited from pre-colonial times. This is helpful when introducing new concepts of development.

4. The old traditions that were detrimental to women's position in the community are being replaced by laws that promote equality between men and women.

5. The marriage law has confirmed women's right in marriage and has done away with polygamy.

6. The ten-household (*dasawisma*) concept.

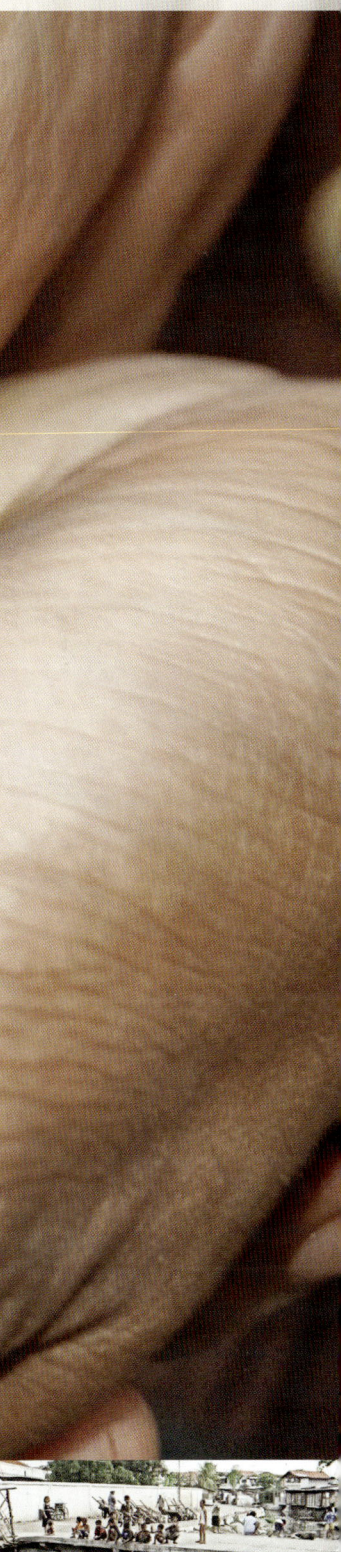

Family Welfare Movement (Pembinaan Kesejahteraan Keluarga - PKK) and its achievements in national development: Indonesia

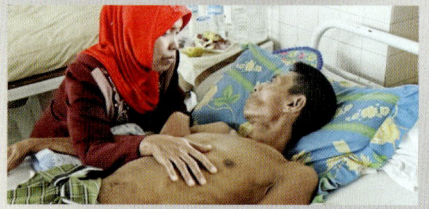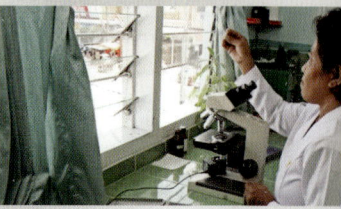

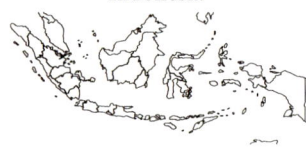
Indonesia

The most significant PKK programme in this respect is its widespread, non-formal education programme

7. Conclusion

Maximum participation by all communities is necessary for sustained national development. Since a family is the smallest unit of society, it is very important to encourage every member of a family to play an active role in developing a happy and prosperous family. This includes mental, spiritual, material and physical well-being. Mothers hold the primary role in a family and therefore, they are central in the development of the family's life. PKK has the duty to urge mothers to play a more active part as vanguards in achieving the goals of family welfare.

Since rural development contributes substantially to national development, PKK has made its contributions through supporting family welfare. The most significant PKK programme in this respect is its widespread, non-formal education programme covering an integrated curriculum training in literacy, primary health care and family planning, managing the Posyandu, teaching civics, caring for the family and community environment, education in home gardening and cloth-making techniques, encouraging mutual help and so forth.

In general, the rural community in Indonesia is dominated by traditional conservative and paternalistic attitudes. These often conflict with the process of women's development. PKK attempts to overcome these problems by improving social communication and convincing women of the advantages of PKK programmes and activities through dasawisma.

Since improving the quality of human development is the basic concept of PKK, its strategy is a bottom–up movement and grass-roots level approach. PKK must expose its members to the fact that development is an integrated process, in which the whole community is developed. PKK is no longer concerned only with economic progress. Therefore, development should be focused on enhancing community capacities for developing their own resources. PKK plays a very important role as a change agent. However, the changes brought about should not disrupt the cultural integrity of rural communities. Though considerable progress has been made by PKK, much remains to be done.

8. Bibliography

Biro Pusat Statistik (Central Bureau of Statistics). *Welfare indicator.* Jakarta: Biro Pusat Statistik, 1985.

Committee on Health Statistics, Southeast Asian Medical Information Centre. *SEAMIC health statistics 1986.* Tokyo: International Medical Foundation of Japan, 1986.

Indonesia, Ministry of Health. *The Third Five-Year Health Development Plan.* Jakarta: Ministry of Health, 1978.

Indonesia, Ministry of Health. *The Fourth Five-Year Health Development Plan.* Jakarta: Ministry of Health, 1983.

Rogers EM, Shoemacher, FF. Communication of innovations, a cross cultural approach. 2nd edition. New York: The Free Press, 1971.

Roestam KS. *Family welfare movement, an alternative for rural women and development.* Proceedings of the CIRDAP Workshop. Quezon City: 1985.

Roestam KS. *Family welfare movement in Indonesia and its achievements.* Jakarta: Family Welfare Movement (PKK), 1985.

Roestam KS. Family welfare movement in Indonesia and its achievements. Jakarta: Family Welfare Movement (PKK), 1987.

Suwandono A. *A study of selected factors influencing the development of primary health care in rural Indonesia – the Banjarnegara experience.* Dissertation presented for the DrPH degree, School of Public Health, University of Hawaii, Honolulu, 1986.

Tim Penggerak Pusat PKK. *Laporan Perkembangan Kegiatan PKK.* Jakarta, 1985.

Yahya S. *Kecendarungan dan Faktor-faktor yang Menpengaruhi Kebijalsanaan Pembangunan Kesehatan.* Jakarta, 1987.

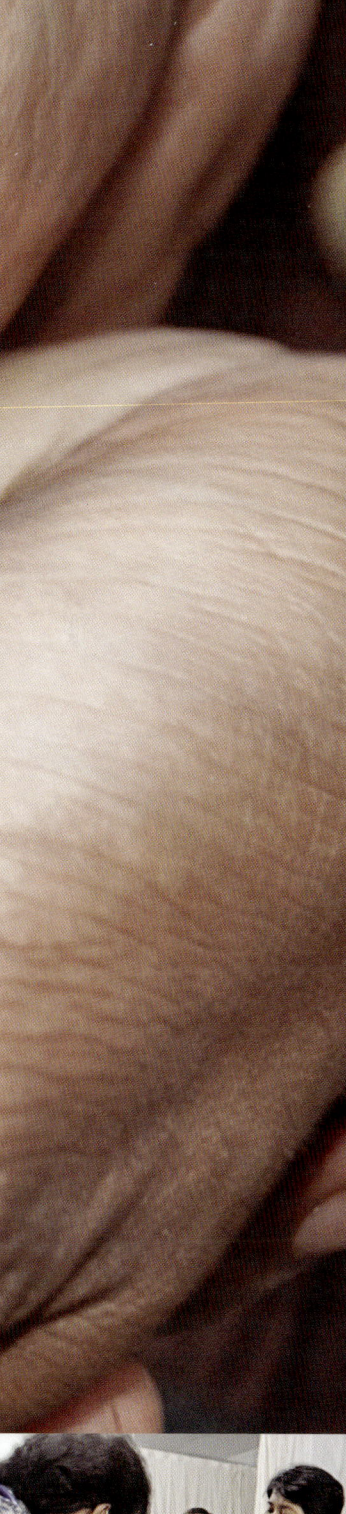

Sasakawa Health Prize: STORIES FROM SOUTH-EAST ASIA

Improving the quality of human development is the basic concept of PKK, its strategy is a bottom-up movement and grass-roots level approach

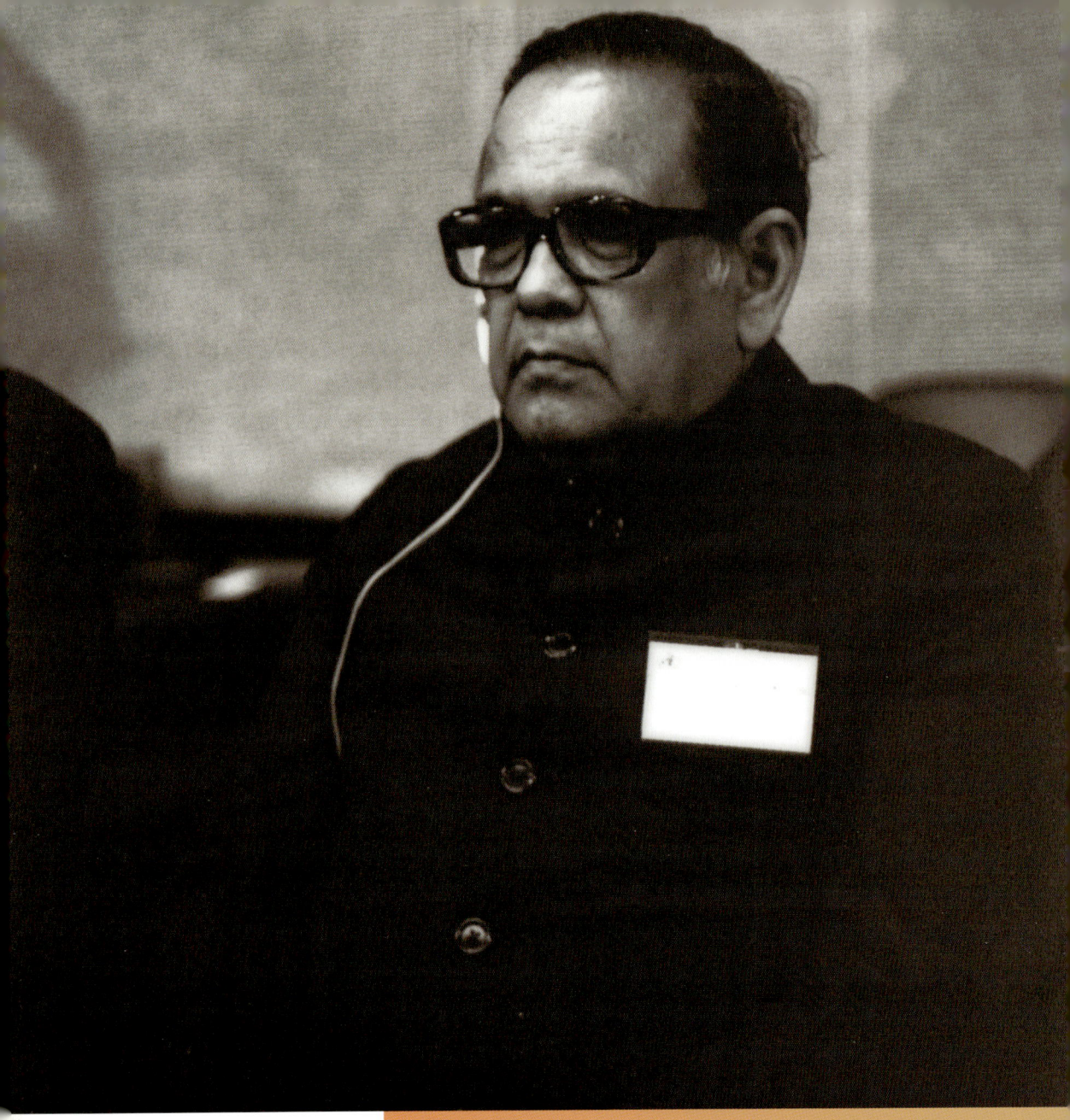

Dr B. N. Tandon, India, Chairman of the Scientific Advisory Committee of the National Institute of Nutrition, Hyderabad, one of the recipients of the 1990 Sasakawa Health Prize.

WHO Photo by Tibor Farkas

CHAPTER 5

1990

Integrated Child Development Scheme (ICDS): India[*]

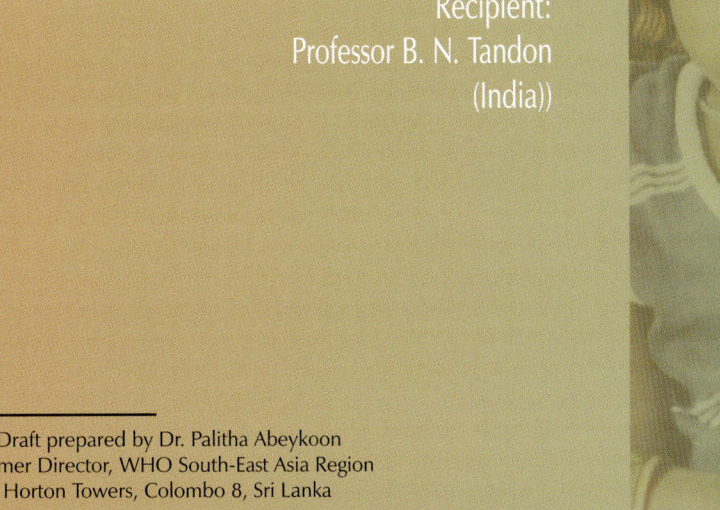

Recipient:
Professor B. N. Tandon
(India))

[*] Draft prepared by Dr. Palitha Abeykoon
Former Director, WHO South-East Asia Region
17, Horton Towers, Colombo 8, Sri Lanka

The Integrated Child Development Scheme (ICDS) was started by the Government of India in 1975. It has been instrumental in improving the health and well-being of mothers and children

1. Summary

The Integrated Child Development Scheme (ICDS) was started by the Government of India in 1975. It has been instrumental in improving the health and well-being of mothers and children below 6 years of age by providing health and nutrition education, health services, supplementary food and preschool education. The ICDS national development programme is one of the largest in the world. It reaches more than 34 million children aged 0–6 years, and 7 million pregnant and lactating mothers. Other programmes that impact on undernutrition include the National Mid-day Meal Scheme, the National Rural Health Mission, and the Public Distribution System (PDS). The challenge for all these programmes and schemes is how to increase their efficiency, impact and coverage.

In the area of child development and nutrition, the United Nations Children's Fund (UNICEF) assists the government to further expand and enhance the quality of ICDS through the following means:

- Improving the training of child-care workers;
- Developing innovative communication approaches with mothers;
- Improving monitoring and reporting systems;
- Providing essential supplies;
- Developing effective community-based early child-care interventions;
- Providing iron–folic acid supplementation to adolescents;
- Providing vitamin A supplementation to children;
- Increasing the use of iodized salt.

2. A coordinated approach to children's health in India: progress report after five years (1975–1980)

2.1 Integrated Child Development Services[1]

Introduction

The Integrated Child Development Services scheme (ICDS) was launched in India on 2 October 1975 as an experimental project in 29 rural and tribal blocks and four urban slums.[2] India has a total of 5011 rural and tribal blocks with approximate populations of 100 000 and 75 000, respectively. The ICDS provides a package of services for children up to six years of age, pregnant women and lactating mothers. Services include immunization, nutrition supplementation (300 additional kcal, 15 g protein, iron, folic acid and vitamin A), nutrition therapy for severely malnourished children, health check-ups, antenatal services, postnatal care, treatment of minor illnesses, preschool education, informal education for women, and health and nutrition education. All services are delivered at a central point in each village (anganwadi) by a local village woman (anganwadi worker) specially trained for this programme. She is an honorary worker and receives a small monthly payment (Rs 125–175; US$ 14–19). The anganwadi receives support and supervision from the health infrastructure (primary health centre) of the block for the health and nutrition programme, and from a child development project officer and staff for social welfare educational services. Faculty members of medical colleges, especially from the departments of paediatrics and community medicine, work for the ICDS as consultants in four capacities – monitoring, evaluation, training and supportive supervision of the workers.

The first report on ICDS indicated the success of the experimental projects.[2] The evaluation of the second phase of ICDS development is reported here. The data have been analysed to find out the impact of the coordinated approach for delivery of health and nutrition services in 1976–80, when the experimental

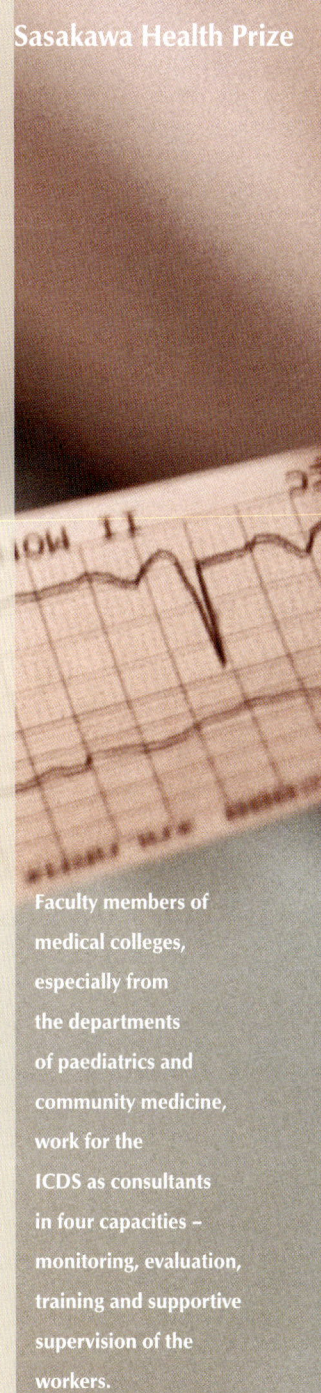

> Faculty members of medical colleges, especially from the departments of paediatrics and community medicine, work for the ICDS as consultants in four capacities – monitoring, evaluation, training and supportive supervision of the workers.

---

[1] Integrated Child Development Service. A coordinated approach to children's health in India. The Lancet. 1981 Mar 21:317(8221): 650-3

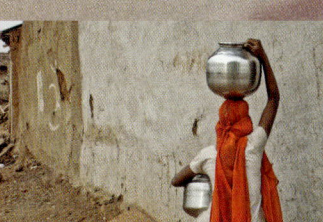

The Integrated Child Development Services scheme (ICDS) was launched in India on 2 October 1975 as an experimental project in 29 rural and tribal blocks and four urban slums

INTEGRATED CHILD DEVELOPMENT SCHEME (ICDS):
INDIA: 1990 (INDIA)

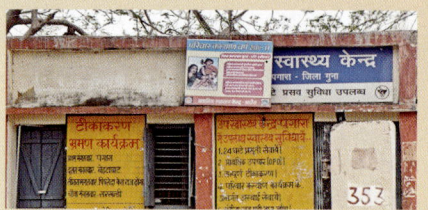
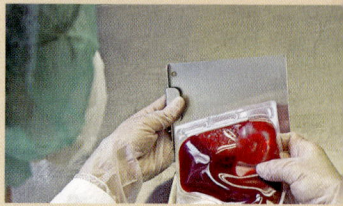

project changed to a national programme to cover a larger population. The rate of change due to ICDS in a year was also estimated by comparing the first and fourth years of the programme. The Government of India has declared it a programme of national importance. It will be expanded to cover 913 of the 5011 community blocks and 87 urban slum areas by 1985.

Subjects and methods

The sample for the study was drawn from 56 ICDS blocks; 23 projects were established in 1975–76 and 33 in 1978–79. The criteria for selection of blocks for ICDS projects have been constant since the scheme began in October 1975. Rural and tribal blocks and urban slums, which are considered backward or underprivileged by the national socioeconomic criteria, are selected for implementation of ICDS. From the revenue records, all the selected villages have similar socioeconomic conditions, with most of the population living below the poverty line; this implies a monthly income for a family of five of less than Rs 300 (US$ 30), which is too low to maintain proper health and nutrition of the family members. Children from the backward classes and with poor nutritional status are registered on a preferential basis at the village centre for ICDS services. Previous studies by the Central Committee for Nutrition and Health in ICDS[3] and the Programme Evaluation Organization of the Planning Commission[4] have confirmed that ICDS services primarily cover poor children from underprivileged socioeconomic groups in the villages.

The sampling methodology for the evaluation study was the same as that of the first.[2] Two serial lists of anganwadis were prepared by village name, one for all anganwadis in villages of the primary health subcentre headquarters, and the other for all anganwadis about 5 km outside the villages of the subcentre headquarters.

Villages with primary healthcentre headquarters were excluded from the above lists. Random samples of the same size were drawn from the two lists. All the households in the sampled anganwadis were surveyed.

> The sample for the study was drawn from 56 ICDS blocks; 23 projects were established in 1975–76 and 33 in 1978–79

The samples studied were as follows:

a. 27,726 preschool children (16 989 rural, 5553 tribal and 5184 urban) in whom a baseline study was conducted before ICDS projects started in 1976.

b. 27,487 preschool children (10 078 rural, 8291 tribal and 9118 urban) whose baseline study was conducted before the ICDS programme started in 1979.

c. 15,882 from the same blocks as sample A, but different children (9266 rural, 3822 tribal and 2794 urban) who were surveyed in 1979–80, about three years after the implementation of ICDS.

d. 10,947 children (5291 rural, 3228 tribal and 2428 urban) from projects established in 1979 were surveyed before the projects began in 1979 and again after one year of ICDS.

e. 2532 children (1552 rural, 570 tribal and 410 urban) were selected from six ICDS projects established in 1976 and surveyed in 1979 and in 1980, i.e. three years and four years after the implementation of ICDS.

In all the populations selected for the study, acceptance was recorded of immunization for BCG, diphtheria, pertussis, tetanus (DPT; 3 doses), and poliomyelitis (3 doses); intervention with supplementary nutrition through a spot-feeding service; distribution of 200 000 IU vitamin A every six months, and health check-ups. Nutritional status was assessed by the weight-for-age method.

Results

Data for samples A and B were studied to find out the percentage of children who accepted immunization and nutrition services, and the nutritional status of the children before the introduction of ICDS programmes in these project areas in 1976 and 1979, respectively (Table 1). These children were receiving services listed separately from those provided by the Department of Health and Social Welfare (DHSW). The percentage receiving BCG immunization fell slightly from 1976 to 1979, whereas the proportion receiving DPT rose in that time (Table

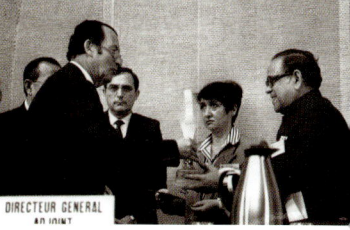

Dr B. N. Tandon, India, receiving the 1990 Sasakawa Health Prize from Professor Plutarco Naranjo, President of the 43rd World Health Assembly.

WHO Photo by Tibor Farkas

Children from the backward classes and with poor nutritional status are registered on a preferential basis at the village centre for ICDS services

INTEGRATED CHILD DEVELOPMENT SCHEME (ICDS):
INDIA: 1990 (INDIA)

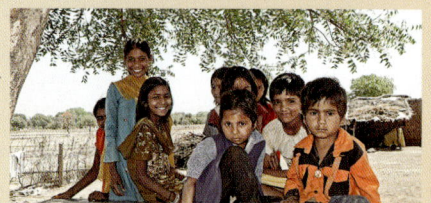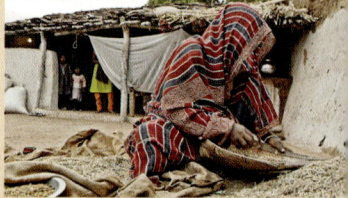

1). Poliomyelitis immunization is not included in the national schedule but in 1979, 9.2% of children received it through an ad-hoc programme. There was an increase in vitamin A administration between 1976 and 1979, but distribution of supplementary nutrition remained almost the same. Severe malnutrition (grades III and IV) decreased from 19.1% in 1976 to 15.1% in 1979.

We next compared data from samples B and C (both surveyed in 1979) to find out whether at that time the services received and the nutritional status of children was better in villages where ICDS had been established for more than three years (sample C) than among children receiving services from elsewhere (Table 1). Both BCG and DPT coverage were higher in three-year-old ICDS blocks (sample C) than in sample B. Health check-ups and distribution of vitamin A and supplementary nutrition were significantly lower in sample B than in sample C. Severe malnutrition was 10.8% in the children receiving services from ICDS compared with 15.1% in the population receiving health and nutrition services from DHSW.

The data for samples A and C (same project blocks but different samples of children) were compared to assess the impact of ICDS three years after its launch. Immunization coverage with BCG and DPT increased by 108% and 622%, respectively, between 1976 (pre-ICDS, sample A) and 1979 (ICDS after three years, sample C). Health check-ups, distribution of vitamin A, and supplementary nutrition showed increases of 221%, 412% and 120%, respectively. Grades III and IV malnutrition declined by 43.5% and grade II malnutrition by 30%.

The final analysis of data from samples D and E aimed to find out whether the rate of change in the receipt of services and in the prevalence of severe malnutrition during the year 1979–80 was greatest in the first or the fourth year of an ICDS programme (Table 2). The rate of change in a year for the acceptance of all the listed services was less in the fourth year of ICDS than in the first year. However, severe malnutrition decreased by almost the same proportion in first-year and fourth-year projects.[5]

> There was an increase in vitamin A administration between 1976 and 1979, but distribution of supplementary nutrition remained almost the same

Table 1: Receipt of essential health services and nutritional status in samples A, B and C

	% of children		
	Sample A (76*)	Sample B (79–80$)	Sample C (79–80#)
Immunization services from	DHSW	DHSW	ICDS
BCG	21.0	17.4	43.6
DPT	4.9	14.0	35.4
Poliomyelitis	NR	9.2	NR
Health check-up	18.5@	15.3	61.3 (57.7@)
Vitamin A	10.3@	17.7	57.1 (52.7@)
Supplementary nutrition	25.2	26.0	55.5
Nutritional status:			
Normal+grade I	47.2	56.2	62.7
Grade II	27.0	28.2	26.2
Grades III+IV	19.1	15.1	10.8
NR	6.7	0.5	0.3

*27 726 children: 23 projects (12 rural, 7 tribal, 4 urban)
$ 27 487 children: 33 projects (12 rural, 12 tribal, 9 urban)
# 15 882 children: same projects as sample A
@ Data for four urban projects not included
NR not recorded

INTEGRATED CHILD DEVELOPMENT SCHEME (ICDS):
INDIA: 1990 (INDIA)

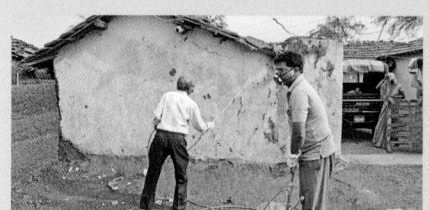
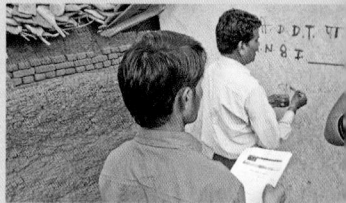

Differences between the samples are significant (P<0.001) except those between A and B in the area of supplementary nutrition (P>0.05) and nutritional status grade II (P<0.01); and that between A and C in nutritional status grade II (P>0.05).

	Fourth year projects*			First year projects#		
	% of children		Rate of change%	% of children		Rate of change
	1979	1980		1979	1980	
Immunization:						
BCG	50.8	65.2	28.3	14.8	26.9	81.8
DPT	33.2	57.3	72.6	8.9	30.4	241.6
Poliomyelitis	15.6	19.5	25.0	5.3	17.0	220.7
Health check-up	58.7	67.7	15.3	12.1	40.9	238.0
Vitamin A	63.6	70.6	11.0	13.8	42.0	204.3
Supplementary nutrition	39.0	55.4	42.0	21.2	34.3	61.8
Nutritional status:						
Normal+grade I	58.2	58.3	0.17	54.4	59.0	8.5
Grade II	28.2	32.3	14.5	29.0	29.0	0.0
Grades III+IV	13.0	9.3	-28.5	16.1	11.8	-26.7
NR	0.2	0.1	..	0.5	0.2	..

Table 2: Rate of change in receipt of health services and nutritional status in first- and fourth-year ICDS project areas

*2532 children: 6 projects (3 rural, 2 tribal, 1 urban)
10 947 children: 20 projects (9 rural, 7 tribal, 4 urban)
NR not recorded

Discussion

The first report on ICDS (March 1981) indicated that this coordinated approach successfully delivered services and improved the nutritional status of the children.[2] By March 1982, a total of 300 projects was sanctioned. The Prime Minister of India announced a 20-point programme[6] on 14 January 1982: ICDS was included as one of the points and it thus became an important national programme. The government decided to expand the programme to 913 rural and tribal blocks (of 5011) and to 87 urban slum projects by the end of 1985. These would cover approximately 20% of the preschool population, and pregnant and lactating women. In fact, this would make it possible to reach 50% or more of the population groups that live below the poverty line and are in greatest need of ICDS services. Owing to financial constraints and the time required for organization, training and assembly of equipment, the ICDS approach has not yet been expanded to cover preschool children of the whole nation.

This study shows that the ICDS approach of the Government of India has continued to be successful as a national programme, with expansion to 300 projects from the original 33 projects. All the parameters for acceptance of health and nutrition services evaluated after four years in the same ICDS project areas showed a significant improvement and there was a decline in the prevalence of severe malnutrition. There was no additional income-raising activity in the villages and slums where these projects had been implemented, which could account for this improvement in the nutritional status of the children. The proportion of India's population below the poverty line has not shown any noticeable change between 1976 and 1980, although accurate data on this point are not available. Improvement in health and nutrition in ICDS blocks therefore cannot be attributed to changes in the economic status of the families.

> ICDS approach of the Government of India has continued to be successful as a national programme, with expansion to 300 projects from the original 33 projects

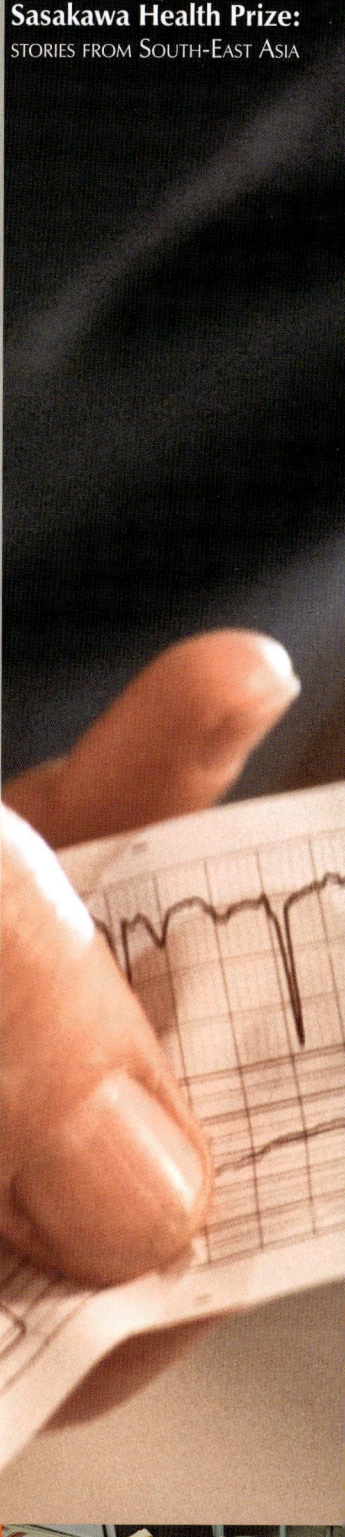

Integrated Child Development Scheme (ICDS):
India: 1990 (India)

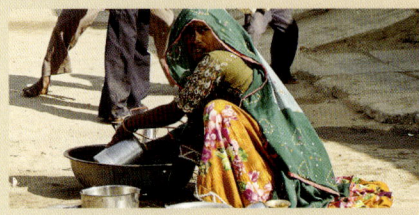 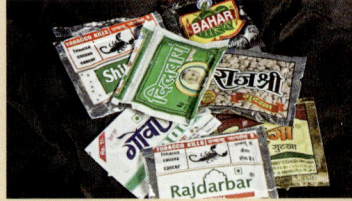

Acceptance of immunization and nutrition services at one point in time (1979) was better among children who had been covered by ICDS for three years (sample C) than in children receiving services independently from DHSW (sample B).

The two populations from which samples B and C were drawn are comparable in their socioeconomic status, according to the criteria laid down for selection of ICDS projects.

It is interesting to note that the non-integrated programme of the health department during 1976–79 was also fairly effective in improving the rates of DPT immunization and distribution of prophylactic vitamin A, and in reducing the prevalence of severe malnutrition. However, these changes were significantly smaller than those that can be achieved through an integrated approach to delivery of health care, nutrition and preschool education.

It has often been stated that the cost of the ICDS approach is high. Establishment of centres in villages, with a voluntary worker in each village, leads to an extra cost of approximately Rs 12 (US$ 1.20) per beneficiary per year, over and above the cost of the health services infrastructure. It is difficult to calculate accurately the additional cost of the village centre for health and nutrition services only, since the centre also provides preschool education for children, and health and nutrition education and functional literacy to the women of the villages. In fact, nearly three quarters of the time of the anganwadi worker at the village centre is spent on these activities. The slight increase in the cost of health and nutrition services needed to establish the village-level centre is not only justified by the results, but seems necessary to ensure better performance of the health infrastructure established at substantial cost in India.

The ICDS approach is a step forward towards decreasing morbidity and mortality in preschool children in India, and to give them the opportunity for optimum growth and development

Sasakawa Health Prize:
STORIES FROM SOUTH-EAST ASIA

The ICDS approach is a step forward towards decreasing morbidity and mortality in preschool children in India, and to give them the opportunity for optimum growth and development. However, immunization coverage (which increased from 21% to 43.6% for BCG and from 4.9% to 35.4% for DPT) must be further improved, and severe malnutrition (which fell from 19.11% to 10.8%) needs to be further reduced. A proportion of children remained unimmunized and malnourished: they did not benefit through ICDS for several reasons, such as non-acceptance of immunization by the parents, lack of safe drinking water in the villages which led to frequent intestinal infections, and interruption in feeding programmes due to difficulties in transporting nutritious food to villages with poor roads. All these factors are receiving special attention, and it is hoped that the goal of Health for All by the year 2000 in India will be achieved earlier than the target date for children and mothers through ICDS.

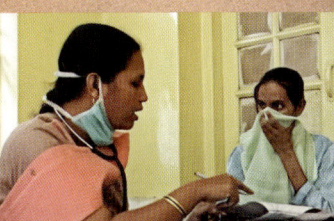

A proportion of children remained unimmunized and malnourished: they did not benefit through ICDS for several reasons, such as non-acceptance of immunization by the parents

INTEGRATED CHILD DEVELOPMENT SCHEME (ICDS):
INDIA: 1990 (INDIA)

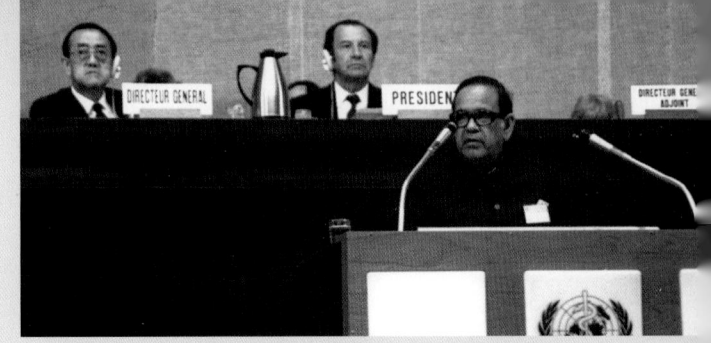

Dr B. N. Tandon, India, recipient of the 1990 Sasakawa Health Prize addressing the 43rd World Health Assembly.
WHO Photo by Tibor Farkas

Consultants for survey teams : Dr Ashok Das, Dr V. K. Karan, Dr J. S. Anand, Dr Vijay Kumar, Dr S. C. Sood, Dr S. K. Rana, Dr M. B. Kanvi, Dr M. G. Javeli, Dr S. K. Behra, Dr K. N. Aggarwal, Dr B. K. Garg, Dr M. K. Chakraborty, Dr Y. L. Vasudeva, Dr K. Indira Bai, Dr B. N. Goswami, Dr Sunder Lal, Dr G. M. Dhar, Dr M. K. Vasundhara, Dr T. Rajagopal, Dr V. Krishnan, Dr M. Zaheer, Dr B. C. Srivastava, Dr K. C. Rajagopalan, Dr Harendra Pratap, Dr S. C. Baldev Raj, Dr Manikyaraju, Dr K. G. Kamala, Dr S. A. H. Zaidi, Dr J. K. Bhatnagar, Dr S. C. Banerjee, Dr Gopal Sharan, Dr T. B. Prasad, Dr D. S. Dave, Dr Y. Srihari Rao, Dr J. N. Khargharia, Dr A. C. Patowary, Dr H. K. Gaur, Dr S. K. Sharma, Dr G. A. Panse, Dr D. Roy, Dr Z. K. Muana, Dr B. Rath, Dr S. K. Debata, Dr R. N. Singh, Dr R. P. Bhattacharjee, Dr Y. C. Mathur, Dr D. N. Shah, Dr M. S. Dattal, Dr B. K. Mahajan, Dr B. Bhandari, Dr S. K. Sen, Dr S. K. Dixit, Dr U. J. Modi, Dr Lalita Bahl, Dr Anand Tate, Dr T. P. Jain, Dr S. Bramhanandam, Dr T. M. V. Prasad Rao, Dr H. Singh, Dr A. B. Desai, Dr V. N. Karandikar, Dr Manju Rastogi, Dr G. P. Mathur, Dr Sitesh Ray, Dr Madhuri Basu, Dr Renu B. Patel, Dr S. U. Warerkar, Dr V. Seth, Dr Jayam Subramaniam, Dr K. Haldar.

Data were analysed at the Biostatistics Division of ICDS Central Cell by Professor K. Ramachandran, Mr B. S. Parmar and Mr Ajit Sahai.

3. References

4. Integrated Child Development Service. A coordinated approach to children's health in India. Lancet. 1981; i: 650–653.

5. Integrated Child Development Services Scheme. New Delhi: Department of Social Welfare, Government of India, 1975.

6. Tandon BN, Ramachandran K, Bhatnagar S. Integrated child development services in India: objectives, organization and baseline survey of the project population. Indian Journal of Medical Research. 1981; 73: 374–384.

7. India, Planning Commission. Evaluation report of the Integrated Child Development Scheme. New Delhi, 2009. http://planningcommission.nic.in/reports/peoreport/peo/peo_icds.pdf - accessed 11 November 2011.

8. Tandon BN, Ramachandran K, Bhatnagar S. Integrated child development services in India: evaluation of the delivery of nutrition and health services and the effect on the nutritional status of the children. Indian Journal of Medical Research. 1981; 73: 385–394.

9. India, Ministry of Information and Broadcasting. The new 20-point programme declaration by the prime minister of India, 14 January, 1982. New Delhi: Directorate of Advertising and Visual Publicity, 1982.

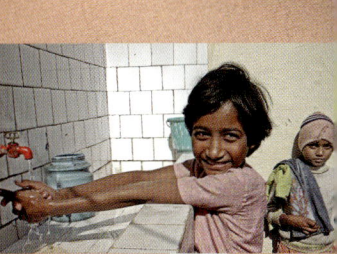

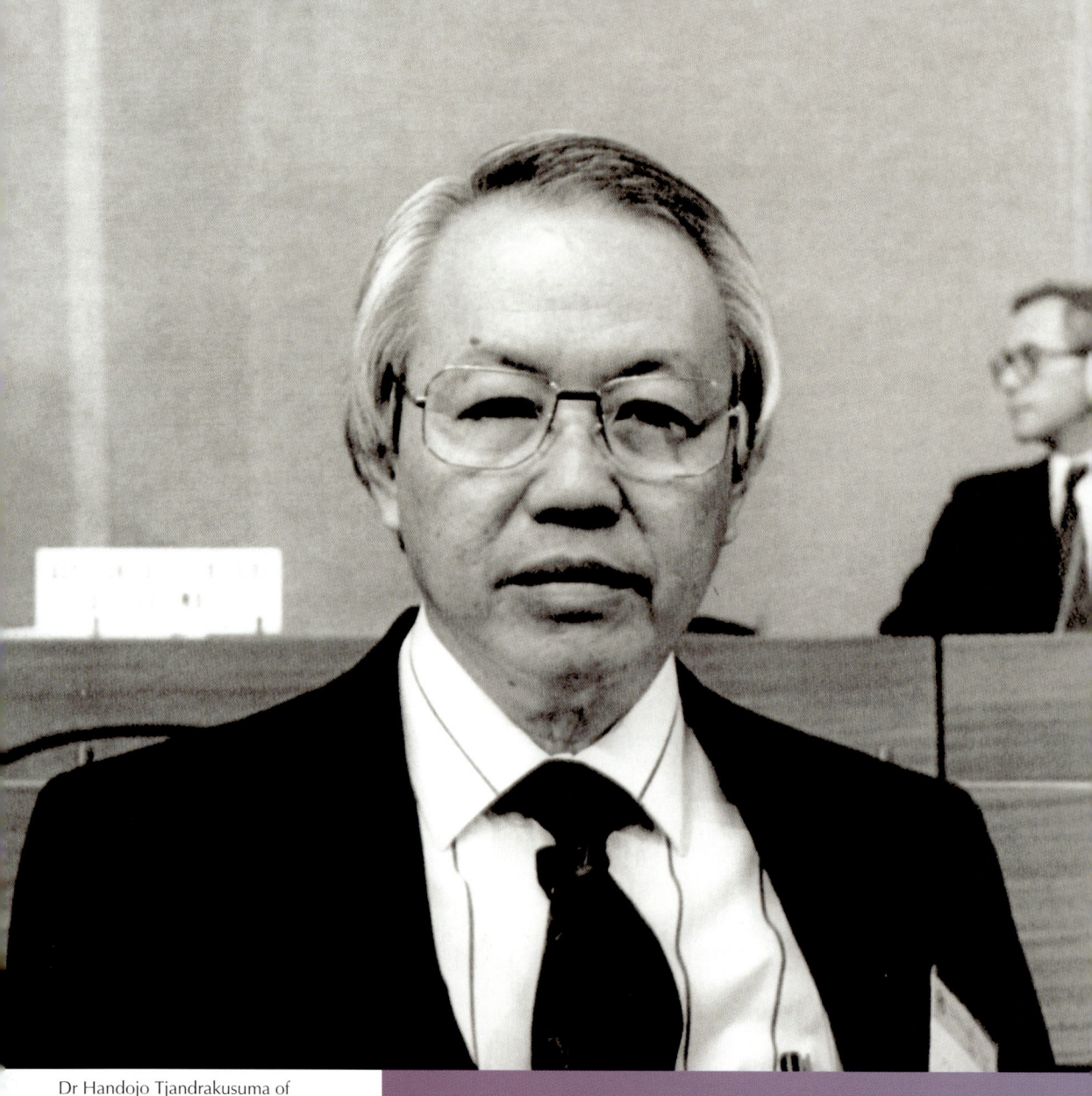

Dr Handojo Tjandrakusuma of Indonesia, one of the winner of the 1992 Sasakawa Health Prize.

WHO Photo by Tibor Farkas

CHAPTER 6

1992

Community-based rehabilitation: improving the quality of life of people with less ability[*]

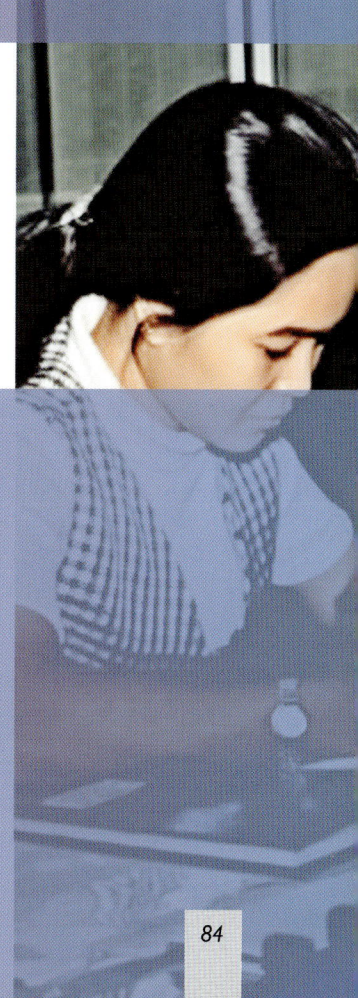

Recipient:
Dr Handojo Tjandrakusuma
(Indonesia)

---

[*] Drafted by Dr Handojo Tjandrakusuma
Former Director of the Community Based Rehabilitation Development and Training Center (CBR-DTC) PPRBM Prof.Dr.Soeharso – YPAC Nasional Jl.LU.Adi Sucipto KM-7 Colomadu-Solo 57176 Indonesia

D r Handojo Tjandrakusuma graduated in 1965 from the Medical Faculty of Airlangga University, Surabaya, Indonesia. Since then, he has been involved in diverse activities related to disability issues

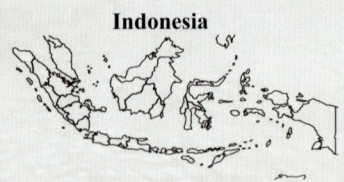

Indonesia

1. Introduction

Dr Handojo Tjandrakusuma graduated in 1965 from the Medical Faculty of Airlangga University, Surabaya, Indonesia. Since then, he has been involved in diverse activities related to disability issues.

Dr Handojo started his career in 1966 at the Rehabilitation Centre (RC) in Surakarta, Central Java. Since 1965, Dr Handojo also held the post of Director of the Academy of Physiotherapy (Ministry of Health) in his hometown Surakarta, Indonesia. In 1970, he attended the WHO Upgrading Course on Medical Rehabilitation in Lebanon. In 1972, under the umbrella of the Children's Rehabilitation Foundation of Indonesia, Dr Handojo founded the Council for Cerebral Palsy (CP) in Indonesia and became its first Director.

Dr Handojo realized that institution-based services at that time did not reach people in the rural areas for various reasons. Poverty prevented people in rural areas from travelling to the rehabilitation centre and institutions located mostly in big cities. Therefore, he started a programme to develop rehabilitation activities in rural areas, which directly involved communities. This programme was called the Village Rehabilitation Programme. The World Health Organization launched a similar concept named Community Based Rehabilitation (CBR) in 1976. Since the WHO concept of CBR was internationally accepted by governments and communities, in 1984, the Council for CP was renamed the CBR Development and Training Centre. Dr Handojo then expanded the CBR strategies to fit the social, cultural and economic situation of the society.

Poverty prevented people in rural areas from travelling to the rehabilitation centre and institutions located mostly in big cities

2. Background of the project

2.1 Community- and institution-based programmes

The motivation behind the proposed strategy was the inaccessibility of current rehabilitation programmes to rural communities. Indonesia consists of 17 667 islands with a population of 237 million; 80% lives in rural areas. In 1977, Dr Handojo mapped the houses of CP patients who sought help at the Children's Rehabilitation Foundation, Surakarta and a larger area. He found that institution-based rehabilitation programmes did not reach a large number of disabled people.

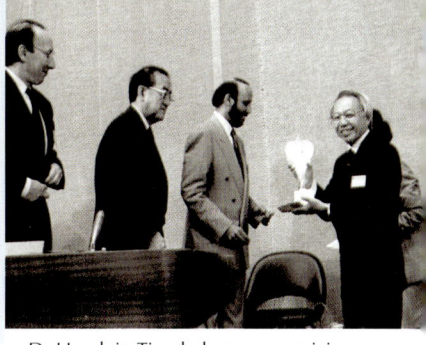

Dr Handojo Tjandrakusuma receiving the 1992 Sasakawa Health Prize from Mr A. Al-Badi, President of the 45th World Health Assembly.

WHO Photo by Tibor Farkas

Traditionally, rehabilitation services have been primarily institutional in nature, located in the cities, and reach only those who live close to the centres. In the institution-based rehabilitation (IBR) model, the responsibility for rehabilitation rests with the disabled persons themselves. In order to avail of the services, however, people with less ability should first be aware of the facilities and services available, and second, be able to access these. In other words, IBR services were waiting for customers to come to them instead of reaching out to customers.

Many disabled people did not understand that rehabilitation services could help them and were not aware that such services existed

There were challenges within this model. The first challenge was that many disabled people did not understand that rehabilitation services could help them and were not aware that such services existed. Second, disabled people did not know where to access these services. Third, they did not even know what kind of help they needed.

Another approach was to extend the IBR services closer to the community. This extension would allow professionals to enter the communities and increase their understanding of disabled people's needs as a part of the community. However, in such a scenario, rehabilitation services were only essentially delivered in the community. There was no community participation or community involvement in the rehabilitation process itself. The CBR approach uses the community as one of the resources for the rehabilitation of people with less ability, as well as resources from IBR.

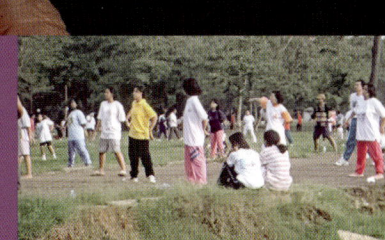

Traditionally, rehabilitation services have been primarily institutional in nature, located in the cities, and reach only those who live close to the centres

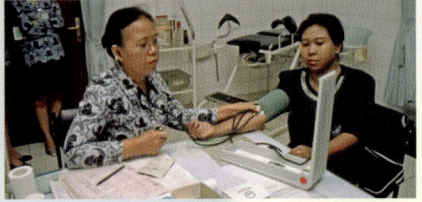
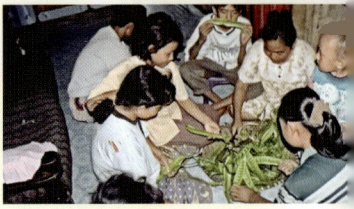

2.2 Defining the ideal CBR model

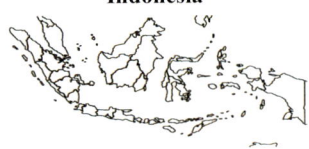

Indonesia

It was not that rehabilitation services did not exist at that time in Indonesia. In fact, there were a number of government and nongovernment departments, agencies and organizations, as well as formal community activities in health care. This was important to consider when examining the availability of resources for the expansion of CBR activities. The Departments of Health, Social Affairs and Education had existing programmes that assisted disabled people in various ways. In addition to these government programmes, there were nongovernmental organizations (NGOs) which supplemented these services. They were responsible for running special schools and training centres for the blind, deaf and mentally challenged, rehabilitation centres specializing in orthopaedic conditions, etc.

A framework of the CBR concept and strategy that was effective and easy to understand would be very useful as a guideline for participating agencies/parties and the community to coordinate and implement CBR programmes together

Coverage of services for disability prevention and rehabilitation needed to be expanded. However, an increase in only the government and nongovernment services would not be effective because the community's awareness and involvement would be minimal. Before any expansion, community sectors should first be empowered in order to "catch up" with existing disability prevention and rehabilitation services. Once the community had used the available resources to their fullest potential, all sectors could expand together. In this way, service expansion would be much more effective and efficient.

A great deal of effort was involved in changing community behaviour (attitude, knowledge and skills). These changes enabled community members to have a better understanding of disability issues (socioeconomic, sociocultural, medical, psychological, etc.), provide a positive environment (physical, psychological, sociocultural and economic) and be responsible for improving the quality of life of people with less ability. CBR was a community development programme in the field of disability prevention and rehabilitation.

Implementation of CBR required the participation of numerous sectors of society with various degrees of knowledge and experience, both professional and non-professional. It must be emphasized that the CBR model or framework should consider the multifaceted contribution of all the different participants.

As a result, the CBR model and concepts should be easily understood by all the participants. This is the only strategy where professionals and non-professionals can work together in a CBR programme. A framework of the CBR concept and strategy that was effective and easy to understand would be very useful as a guideline for participating agencies/parties and the community to coordinate and implement CBR programmes together.

CASE 1

Slamet and the homemade tofu production house

In 1988, Slamet, who had a speech and hearing problem, was very happy when Mr Joko from CBR Surakarta and the village community of District Klaten found him a job as a production staff at a local homemade tofu production house.

After assessing the practical, health and safety aspects, the owner of the factory was happy to employ Slamet. However, it was not as easy as expected. The owner and colleagues had trouble in communicating information to him. Since there was no one in that village with professional experience and skills in dealing with disability, the owner then invited Mr Joko as an adviser to find a solution to the communication problem.

With time, patience and commitment, Slamet was successfully able to fit in with the factory life. He was able to complete his tasks and ineract socially with other workers. He was treated in the same manner as the other workers. After two years, Slamet was still happily working in that tofu factory and became an asset to the company.

Slamet and the owner of the tofu home industry had empowered themselves to take a decision. They did not rely on outside assistance in running their day-to-day activities. Therefore, CBR is a process by, for and with the community.

The case study above shows that a local community was able to identify the needs of a disabled person. Within a local community members should be able to discover their own method of rehabilitation. In CBR, the community should identify a disabled person's needs by itself, and fulfil these with locally available resources.

Sasakawa Health Prize:
STORIES FROM SOUTH-EAST ASIA

The Departments of Health, Social Affairs and Education had existing programmes that assisted disabled people in various ways. In addition to these government programmes, there were nongovernmental organizations (NGOs) which supplemented these services

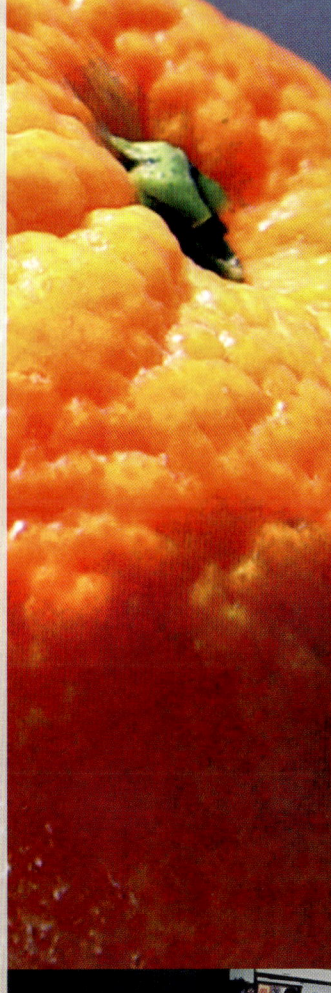

Community-based
rehabilitation: improving the
quality of life of people with
less ability: 1992 (Indonesia)

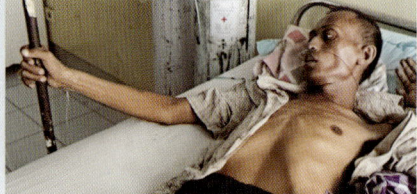 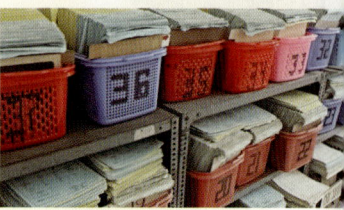

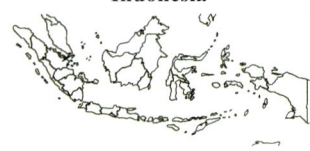
Indonesia

CBR is not just a way to help people with less ability. It is also a process of empowerment, which enables community members, including people with less ability, to cooperatively participate in their own decision-making process. The community is involved in deciding its own needs, rather than having ideas imposed on them from the outside. This feature is critical for understanding the "real" CBR. Those who wish to be implementers of CBR must only introduce the idea of CBR and then permit the villagers to determine what the idea meant to them and how best it could be used in their community. This concept is about community development in the field of disability prevention, rehabilitation and improvement in the quality of life.

3. Strategic thinking

3.1 Behavioural change in the community

The CBR model was explained to the community using the analogy of a house. CBR could be conceptualized as a house with a base and three pillars supporting a roof. The base consisted of the concept and philosophy of CBR. The first pillar consisted of local village members, the second pillar of trained volunteers or CBR cadres. The third pillar consisted of professionals and institutions. It was important to recognize that all three pillars were necessary within the CBR model because all these resources had important contributions to make in the successful implementation of CBR. The community with its potential was the main agent responsible and was the main resource for programme implementation. The programme must be relevant to community needs and based on resources from within the community.

Any person or organization who wants to implement CBR is in fact a "change agent". Behaviour change in the community only occurs when a "change agent" effectively introduces new knowledge and skills that contribute to positive changes in the community. The objective of the changes is that the community can reach a certain behaviour level that supports disability prevention and rehabilitation activities.

> CBR is not just a way to help people with less ability. It is also a process of empowerment, which enables community members, including people with less ability, to cooperatively participate in their own decision-making process

Case 2 below shows that CBR is a method to improve the quality of life. Mrs Dyah, a CBR cadre, realized that a disabled person had the same needs as a non-disabled person. Case 2 is about the human need to have a family. A CBR cadre of a community is a community member who has the right attitude towards disability issues and is able to change the behaviour of the local community.

> Integrated programme should obtain the full support and involvement of the higher levels

CASE 2

The change agent – quality of life of people with less ability

In 1989, 27-year-old Mulyono from village Plumbon, Mojolaban, Central Java wanted to marry a woman from his village. He suffered from polio. According to Javanese culture, a man who would like to marry a woman should send his proposal to the future bride's parents to obtain permission and fulfil the terms and conditions of the traditions.

The mother of the future bride did not accept the proposal because of his physical condition. The people from the village believed that his condition could be passed on to the next generation. Fortunately, after long counselling from Mrs Dyah, the wife of village leader and a CBR cadre from that community, she accepted the proposal. Mrs Dyah found that generally, rejection and a wrong perception of disability by the villagers was caused by the lack of knowledge of disabilities.

Mrs Dyah was a change agent within her community and successfully introduced new knowledge that resulted in community acceptance towards a disabled person. Until today, Mulyono lives happily with his wife and three healthy children.

3.2 The framework

Various disability prevention and rehabilitation activities take place in the community and they depend on the abilities and resources of those who perform them. Referring to the "house and three pillars" analogy, it is possible to consider the performance of CBR activities in three groups. Every pillar has technical and managerial aspects.

The technological activities were aimed at the grass-roots level community members who were provided with knowledge and skills that they would employ in practical ways. Early detection and early intervention for disability were examples of technical activities. In other words, CBR cadres provided the technical activities of CBR.

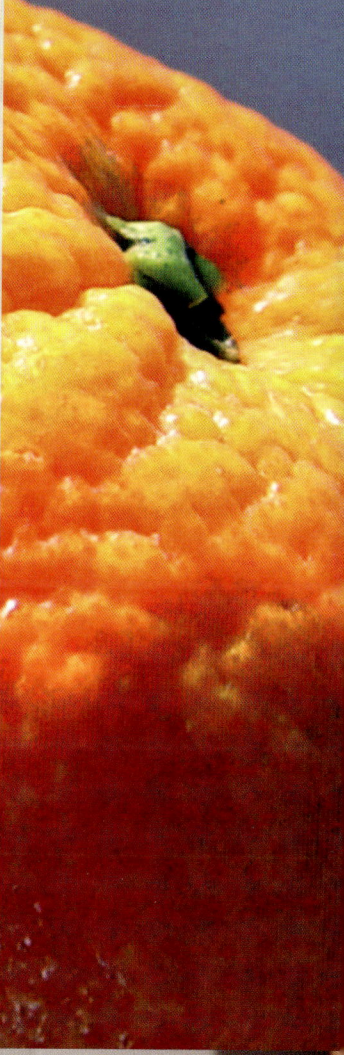

Community-based rehabilitation: improving the quality of life of people with less ability: 1992 (Indonesia)

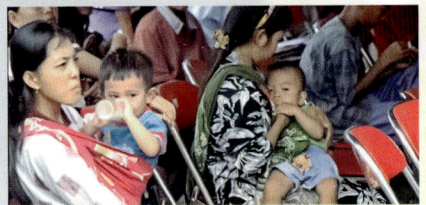
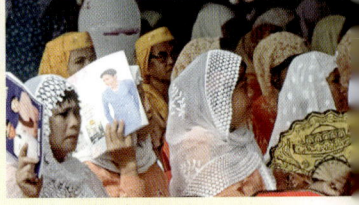

Indonesia

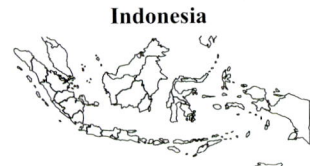

Various disability prevention and rehabilitation activities take place in the community and they depend on the abilities and resources of those who perform them

Those in the community who were active in the local government and institutions were employed in organizational/managerial capacities. Local government personnel formed a "CBR coordinating team". The purpose of this body was to manage activities such as developing and administering financial resources and organizing disability reassessment days.

The contributions to CBR made by the community, CBR cadres and professionals were all equally valuable. It could be seen that this traditional concept of rehabilitation did not fully reflect the integrated way in which the community, trained members of that community (i.e. CBR cadres) and professionals all cooperated and integrated their skills in such a way that all contributed to community-based rehabilitation. The "right way" of understanding CBR was to recognize that CBR was an open system with important contributions by diverse persons and organizations along the "professional–non-professional" continuum.

3.3 Integration of CBR with available resources

The first strategic issue was how the new CBR programme could be specifically incorporated into pre-existing community activities. It was too expensive and complicated to develop a separate infrastructure for community-based disability prevention and rehabilitation. The second strategic issue was to select an effective entry programme. Effective entry programmes should be easy to implement, have visible results and be easy to integrate into existing programmes. One benefit of an effective programme would be the inclusion of both technical and motivational aspects, i.e. develop community interest in disability problems. Therefore, it was suggested to develop CBR activities that could be easily integrated into the existing system. It was also beneficial to attach CBR services to programmes which had national high priority such as primary health care and nutrition programmes.

From the inception of any CBR implementation programme, its sustainability must also be considered. Too often, continuity is not considered until the very late stages (once the support and resources of the initiators are removed).

Sasakawa Health Prize:
Stories from South-East Asia

Programme maintenance must be considered right in the beginning so that every effort can be made to sustain the programme throughout the implementation process. The CBR programme should include orientation of the community in the contingency plan so that it can have some responsibility in maintaining the programme. Otherwise, there is a real danger that CBR activities may fail.

Several techniques for CBR maintenance were used and proposed. Because CBR programmes had already become a part of routine community activities and government services, a reporting and recording system was included in the existing routine. Reminder programmes were used to continue CBR presence in the villages. These reminders consisted of return visits from CBR implementers, for example, visiting guests from other CBR villages. The presence of international guests at a local village provided significant prestige to the village and motivated the members. In addition, audiovisual presentations such as slide shows and films about rehabilitation and disability were very popular. Another proposed idea was to have an annual "Cadres competition/award".

3.4 Economy and income generation

Income generation is a strategic issue. Vocational rehabilitation was not a part of CBR. The primary reason for this was that vocational rehabilitation was too narrow in its considerations, and often did not focus sufficiently on the economic situation of the community marketplace that the disabled persons would return to.

The focus of CBR implementation should be broader than just the disabilities of a person. It should also include their capability for income generation. The focus must be broadened to include the laws of the marketplace. Without this consideration, the best efforts at vocational training would be lost. In order to survive in the current economic environment, the concept of CBR should also include "income generation".

> The technological activities were aimed at the grass-roots level community members who were provided with knowledge and skills that they would employ in practical ways

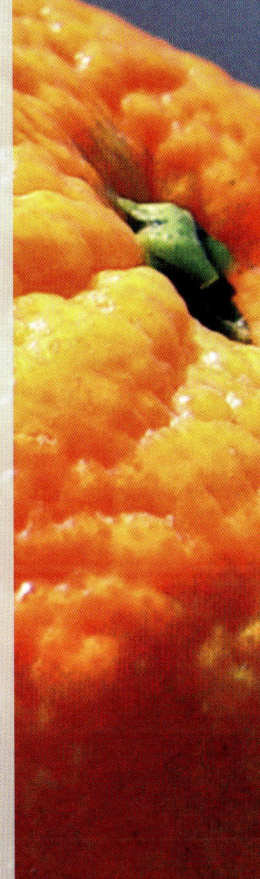

> The Community-based rehabilitation (CBR) programme should include orientation of the community in the contingency plan so that it can have some responsibility in maintaining the programme

Community-based rehabilitation: improving the quality of life of people with less ability: 1992 (Indonesia)

Illustration

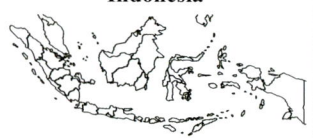
Indonesia

Essential factors for successful income-generating activities

A young paraplegic might have hand function, upper body coordination, as well as an interest in being a barber. He could be trained for this and return to his village to earn his living in this way. On the other hand, he might receive this training and, on return to his village and working for some months relatively successfully, discover that other barbers have just moved into the community. If all of them cannot be supported, the one who succeeds will be the one who can compete best in economic terms. The determination to succeed does not depend upon merit or effort. The success of income-generating programmes depends on just that – generating income.

Vocational rehabilitation was too narrow in its considerations, and often did not focus sufficiently on the economic situation of the community marketplace that the disabled persons would return to

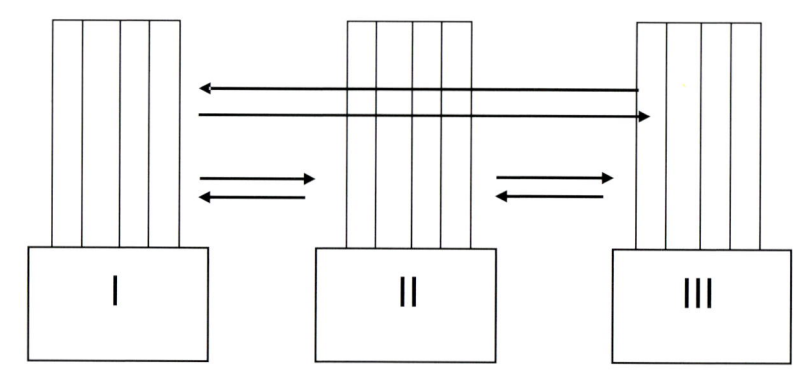

PILLAR I

The community members detect disability and raise funds for the necessary treatment (CBR activities done by community members in general=mothers)

PILLAR II

Organize training programme on early detection of disability by community members (CBR activities done by specially trained community members/cadres=women's organization)

PILLAR III

Develop a manual for ED of disability, organize training for trainers, diagnose cases and provide referral services (CBR activities done by professionals/institutions=puskesmas & posyandu)

The Illustration above indicates the other essential elements required to rehabilitate disabled people by providing them with life skills to earn in the community. Skills training that was suitable for the person's condition was not the main success factor for generating income. More importantly, a careful assessment of the actual economic situation, and family and CBR cadre support determined success in generating income.

4. Case studies

4.1 Early Detection of Disabilities Programme in 18 villages

From January 1994 to December 1995, early detection (ED) programmes were implemented in 18 villages in the districts of Surakarta, Central Java with funding from the Sasakawa award. Initially, ED had two main sub-programmes – on education and practical activities. To ensure that the programme would be practical and sustainable, CBR Surakarta decided to integrate ED with established government and community programmes. The most suitable programme at that time was the Posyandu (National Mother and Child Health Programme) under Puskesmas (Lower District Clinic).

Integration of the three pillars

Any integrated programme should obtain the full support and involvement of the higher levels. For instance, the Posyandu Mother and Child Programme was under Puskesmas or the Lower District Clinic, and the Lower District Clinic was under the Department of Health. From the sustainability point of view, one of the Puskesmas' activities was to give support to the Posyandu on ED. Integration of the three pillars helped to pool resources, all of which were essential in contributing to the success of the programme.

Integration with the Posyandu

The main ED programmes were education programmes for communities and training programmes for medical staff. The education programme was informative and oriented the target audiences of women's organizations/groups/CBR cadres to ED in the villages. The objective of this strategy was to develop cadres who would be able to pass on this information to other women's organizations/groups, the Posyandu and Puskesmas. Meanwhile, the objectives of training medical staff were that they had the ability to train others, and expand and conduct ED, particularly in the programme villages.

A programme evaluation in November 1995 showed that six Puskesmas had implemented ED with 170 medical staff trained in ED. Although the process was

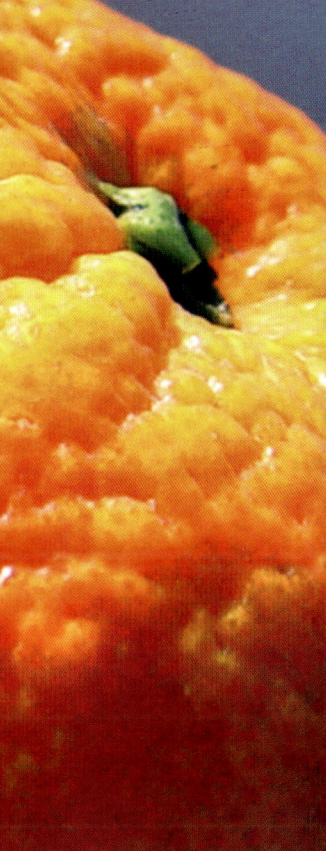

The determination to succeed does not depend upon merit or effort. The success of income-generating programmes depends on just that – generating income

Dr Handojo Tjandrakusuma of Indonesia, one of the winner of the 1992 Sasakawa Health Prize.

WHO Photo by Tibor Farkas

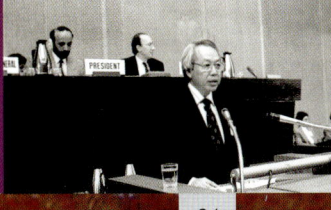

The massive political changes and development of local autonomy rights affected many organizations in Indonesia. Development could also be seen in the areas of communication, transportation and information technology

Community-based
rehabilitation: improving the
quality of life of people with
less ability: 1992 (Indonesia)

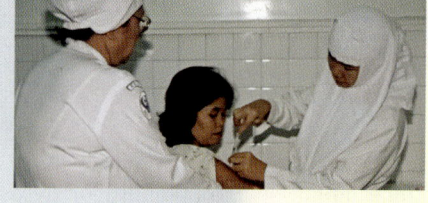 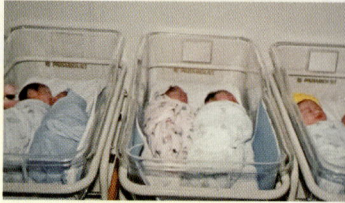

Indonesia

Dr Handojo's specific role in developing CBR programmes led him to receive the Sasakawa Health Prize from WHO in 1992. He is a recognized speaker at various seminars and workshops, both national and international

not as fast as expected, Puskesmas staff members had also started giving training and orientation to cadres at Posyandus. A posyandu in District Klaten even added a counter dedicated to ED and identified 25 cases of late development. As a result, more and more mothers demanded information on ED. ED projects had adopted a suitable method where tangible results could be seen in the targeted area. Knowledge on disability increased significantly in the villages.

4.2 Harelip operations project

In the rural areas, many people did not want to undergo operations because of various factors. such as finances, and a lack of education and information.

In 1995, CBR Surakarta collaborated with government and community organizations on a project called "Operasi bibir sumbing" and hernia in District Tegal. To give other organizations ownership of the disability projects in rural areas, this project involved Pusat Pengembangan dan Latihan Rehabilitasi Para Cacat Bersumberdaya Masyarakat (PPRBM) Surakarta, Social Welfare Department of Tegal, Manunggal Health Organization of Slawi subdistrict Tegal, Women's Association of District Tegal, and the Micro Economy-Anniversary Team of Tegal District. This project targeted 14 poor patients below 15 years of age.

Initially, the society of Tegal reviewed the situation and US$ 375 were raised by all the five organizations along with family contributions. Further, orientation to and implementation of the programmes were done by a team from the Social Welfare of Tegal, Public Hospital of Slawi, Department of Health District Tegal, subdistrict heads and subdistrict puskesmas. In 1996–1997, the collaboration of the third pillar completed the second phase of the project, in which 56 children were successfully operated. As a result, this project successfully restored self-confidence. Parents who were initially afraid of the operation spread the word about the successful operations. This encouraged other parents to have their children operated in the next year's programme. Because of this collaboration, awareness of CBR Surakarta increased in wider areas as well as in the government and community organizations involved. These projects educated not only rural communities but also high-level organizations on their roles in disability. The collaboration of government organizations and NGOs is an example of applying the third pillar in CBR.

5. Conclusion

In 2004, before Dr Handojo resigned from his position as Director of CBR Surakarta, he left behind a concept in relation to community changes. Indonesia was undergoing reformation from 1998 to 2004. The massive political changes and development of local autonomy rights affected many organizations in Indonesia. Development could also be seen in the areas of communication, transportation and information technology. CBR Surakarta realized that most of its strategies were no longer suitable for the community. Therefore, CBR Surakarta altered its strategy to suit the political, economic, social and cultural environment in the community.

6. Epilogue

Dr Handojo's specific role in developing CBR programmes led him to receive the Sasakawa Health Prize from WHO in 1992. He is a recognized speaker at various seminars and workshops, both national and international. As the Director of the CBR Training Centre, with the support of Nippon Foundation and United Nations Economic and Social Commission for Asia and the Pacific (UNESCAP), in 2000, he organized the Asia Pacific Conference on Tourism for People with Disability in Bali, and was chairperson of the conference committee. His work in welfare is well recognized in Indonesia. In 1998, he received the Ministerial Award from the Minister of Social Welfare for pioneering work and outstanding service in social welfare. In 1999, the Indonesia National Council of Welfare appreciated his dedication and work for the welfare of people with disability.

In 2004, he resigned from CBR DTC Training Centre and trained the next director to continue his mission. Dr Handojo is still very active as the chairperson of the boards of several foundations such as the Pantikosala Health Foundation Surakarta, Warga Education Foundation and National Pharmacy Foundation, as well as the main advisor to the Jakarta School of Orthotics and Prosthetics. As the founder and director of RENA Barrier Free Tourism Development Foundation in 1998, he would like to further improve the quality of life of people with disabilities through tourism.

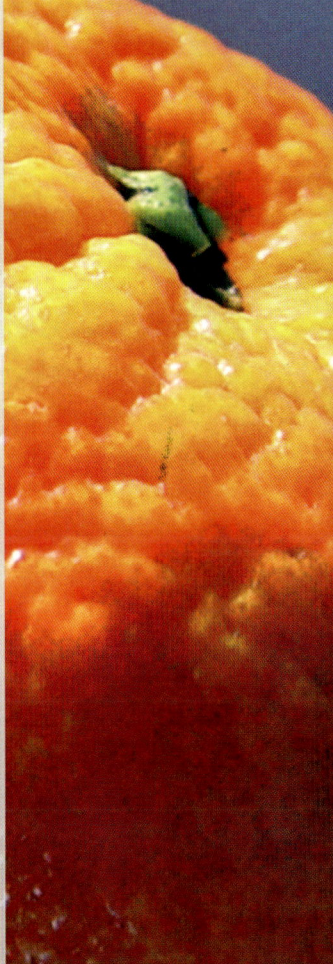

> Projects educated not only rural communities but also high-level organizations on their roles in disability

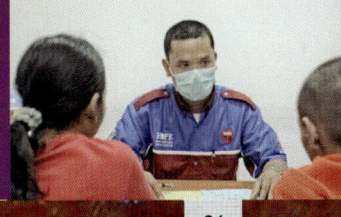

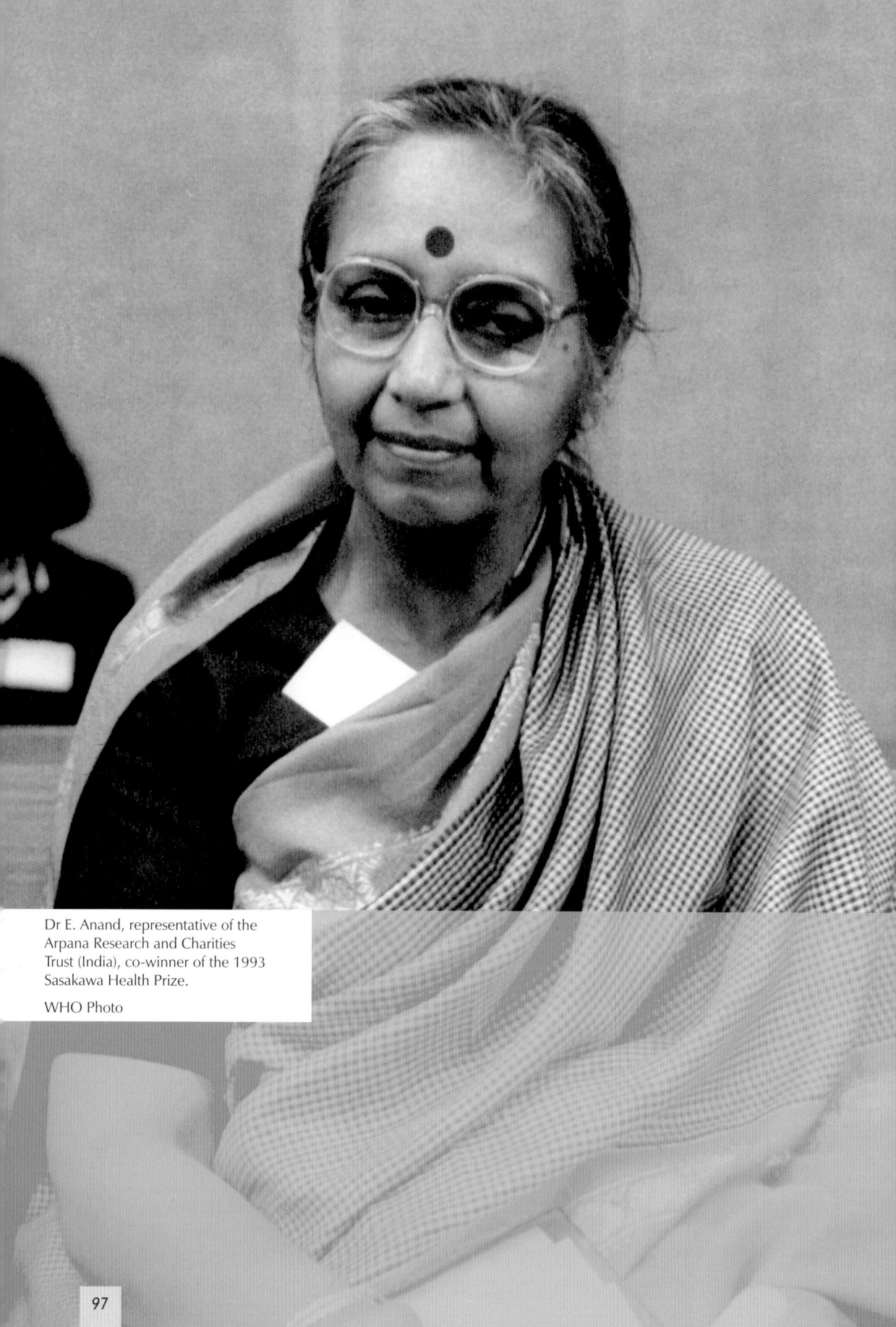

Dr E. Anand, representative of the Arpana Research and Charities Trust (India), co-winner of the 1993 Sasakawa Health Prize.

WHO Photo

CHAPTER 7

1993

Paradigm shift through development programmes in selected villages of Haryana: Arpana Research and Charities Trust–India[*]

Recipient:
Arpana Research and Charities Trust
(India)

[*] Draft prepared by Mrs Anne Robinson and Mrs Aruna Dayal
Arpana Research & Charities Trust, Madhuban, Karnal, Haryana, India

Arpana started in 1980. It built up a broad-based infrastructure for the delivery of primary health care and socioeconomic programmes in its target area of 36 villages in Haryana

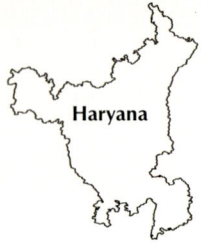

1. Introduction

"Arpana" means dedication. The Arpana family is guided by Param Pujya Ma and consists of some 60 residents from different lands and faiths. They live as one family and comprise people with considerable experience from disciplines such as medicine, law, engineering, education, architecture, economics, social welfare, general management and computers. All are volunteers for life, and live and work among the needy rural people they serve.

The Arpana family is guided by Param Pujya Ma and consists of some 60 residents from different lands and faiths

Arpana started in 1980. It built up a broad-based infrastructure for the delivery of primary health care and socioeconomic programmes in its target area of 36 villages in Haryana. Arpana provided ongoing, in-service training to primary health care workers in these 36 villages. A 75-bed hospital with five major disciplines provided comprehensive health care and was the training centre, referral base and permanent base of operations for the mobile units and delivery of primary health care in these villages.

Each team consisted of a trained midwife, two Integrated Child Development Scheme workers, a male village health worker (VHW) and part-time motivators. The workers also visited other rural health-care projects for new ideas, to increase their confidence and develop linkages with others in the same field.

This health training to workers spread knowledge at a minimal cost and helped to build rapport with the beneficiaries. It was a permanent investment in the future welfare of rural communities. In rural India, with limited trained medical personnel and resources, this is perhaps the most cost-effective and easily replicable method of promoting health care.

Arpana also gave the highest priority to awareness creation of basic health-care principles, preventive health initiatives and community participation to ensure a long-term solution to health and social problems, and to promote well-being in thousands of rural homes.

Sasakawa Health Prize

2. Target areas

The Arpana Trust complex is situated at Madhuban, 11 km outside the town of Karnal in the state of Haryana, and is 114 km north of Delhi.

Haryana: Arpana's target area was 36 villages in Karnal District, with a population of approximately 48 000. Villages with a scarcity of government facilities were selected and all were located within 25 km of the base in Madhuban. Intensive health care was provided through mobile services and a network of VHWs. Villages covered for eye care extended up to 50 km from Madhuban.

Himachal Pradesh: Arpana hospital also served as a training and referral base in Himachal. Arpana had a health-care service in Chamba District, Himachal Pradesh, covering some 160 villages. A mobile service conducted camps in seven village centres to bring them general medical and maternal/child health services. The Medical Centre at Dalhousie was equipped with X-ray and laboratory facilities, and a token two-bed indoor facility.

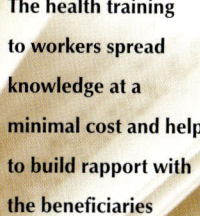

The health training to workers spread knowledge at a minimal cost and helps to build rapport with the beneficiaries

3. Project goals

To improve health and well-being through provision of medical inputs and development initiatives, especially for empowering women.

3.1 General health objectives

1. To reduce infant mortality

2. To improve the nutritional and health status of children below six years of age

3. To reduce maternal mortality and morbidity

4. To prevent blindness and restore sight to the blind in an ever-widening target area.

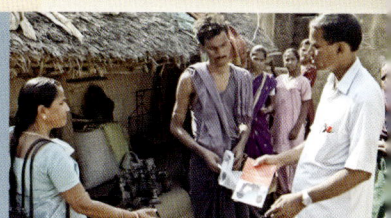

Arpana also gave the highest priority to awareness creation of basic health-care principles, preventive health initiatives and community participation to ensure a long-term solution to health and social problems, and to promote well-being in thousands of rural homes

PARADIGM SHIFT THROUGH DEVELOPMENT PROGRAMMES IN SELECTED VILLAGES OF HARYANA: ARPANA RESEARCH AND CHARITIES TRUST–INDIA: 1993 (INDIA)

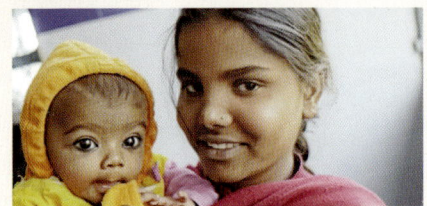
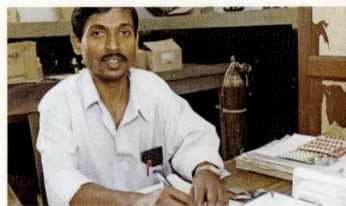
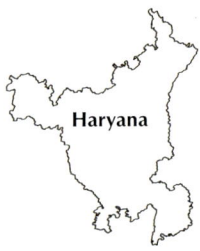

Women are brought up in an environment of neglect, and are considered burdens because of the dowry that parents have to provide at the time of marriage

3.2 General development objectives

1. To raise the standard of living and quality of life of village communities

2. To provide supplemental income for women to ensure that they had food and basics for the family

3. To provide literacy skills and create awareness among women of new and beneficial methods of action

4. To provide a safe and caring environment for preschool children while their mothers were working

5. To stimulate the overall development of children attending the day-care centres

6. To impart knowledge, skills and training to local village midwives, health workers and motivators

7. To increase the level of social awareness, particularly among rural women, and bring about community participation in self-help programmes.

4. Main activities

4.1 Comprehensive approach to primary health care

In rural Haryana, health is a low priority. Women are brought up in an environment of neglect, and are considered burdens because of the dowry that parents have to provide at the time of marriage. A woman is discriminated against for food, clothing and education. Married between the ages of 15 and 17 years, she is unaware of her responsibilities as a wife and mother. In her new home, she is treated with hostility or indifference unless she has a wealthy father or is able to quickly produce a son. From the day she is married, she is expected to work hard as well as give birth to children in quick succession and rear them. In fact, her role in rearing a child seems to be less important than her role in doing

Sasakawa Health Prize:
STORIES FROM SOUTH-EAST ASIA

the many household chores, looking after the milch animals in the house and working in the fields. Children are brought up by their grandmothers or older siblings. Deliveries are carried out by traditional birth attendants (TBAs), who are uneducated and untrained.

It was in this environment that Arpana began its work. The programmes gradually evolved according to their acceptance by the community and availability of funds. The approach varied according to the need.

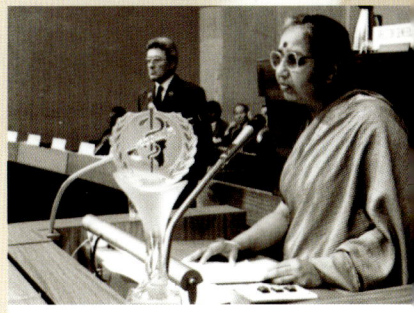

Dr E. Anand, representative of the Arpana Research and Charities Trust (India), co-winner of the 1993 Sasakawa Health Prize, addressing the 46th World Health Assembly.

WHO Photo

The low literacy rate of women made it hard for them to perceive that health problems stem from poor habits of nutrition and hygiene. Women and children lived on the borderline of ill health, and medical care was sought only when an acute health problem arose. No attempt was made to improve the underlying factors of health. The perceived health need was only for curative services. There was no perceived need for mother and child health (MCH) services, which were greatly required.

Deliveries are carried out by traditional birth attendants (TBAs), who are uneducated and untrained

To overcome these problems, the following activities were started:

- *Income generation for women:* by providing handicraft work for women which they could do in their homes, and marketing the handicrafts produced by them.

- *Health services (Arpana Rural Medical Services) at three levels:* a primary level through VHWs and TBAs; a secondary level through mobile clinics and camps; and a tertiary level through a 75-bed hospital with five disciplines.

- *Education ('Arpana Premanjali" programme):* this included education for preschool children; care of children less than three years of age; provision of supplementary nutrition; non-formal education and functional literacy for adolescent girls and women; and child-to-child programmes – schoolchildren who conducted health education and health activities in their own communities.

- *Training:* to produce handicrafts (women and supervisors); in health (health workers, TBAs, and community health workers).

The low literacy rate of women made it hard for them to perceive that health problems stem from poor habits of nutrition and hygiene

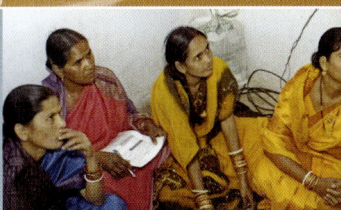

PARADIGM SHIFT THROUGH
DEVELOPMENT PROGRAMMES
IN SELECTED VILLAGES OF
HARYANA: ARPANA RESEARCH
AND CHARITIES TRUST–INDIA:
1993 (INDIA)

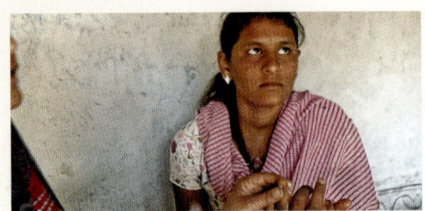
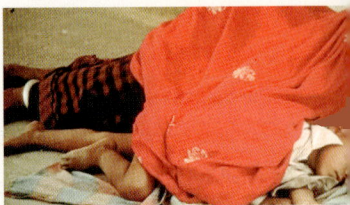

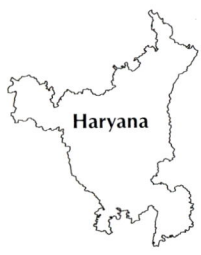

Men and women are selected from the community and trained to conduct health-care activities in the villages

5. Arpana Rural Medical Services (ARMS)

5.1 Methodology and design of referral system for health services

Health services were provided at three levels.

Primary level

Men and women were selected from the community and trained to conduct health-care activities in the villages. TBAs who took care of 70%–80% of childbirths in the villages were untrained. Arpana trained these women and provided them with simple materials for their work, making them a part of the health-care delivery system.

Secondary level

The mobile clinic team consisted of a doctor and /or auxiliary nurse midwife with helpers. This team covered 36 villages, providing skilled support to the primary-level workers who brought referral cases to them. It provided antenatal care, conducted well-baby clinics with immunization, growth monitoring, provided treatment for general ailments and had laboratory facilities.

Tertiary level

Arpana hospital had 75 beds and five disciplines: Medicine, Surgery, Obstetrics and Gynaecology, Ophthalmology and Dentistry. The hospital was the referral base and also where training was imparted to the different cadres of workers. Cases from the secondary level were referred to the base hospital. Serious cases identified in the field were also brought to the hospital by VHWs.

5.2 Health interventions at the primary level

1. *Infectious diseases:* The VHWs learnt to treat minor ailments such as boils, scabies, conjunctivitis, colds and coughs with simple remedies. If patients did not respond, they were referred to the monthly mobile clinic or the referral base hospital. Major infections such as diarrhoea and other gastrointestinal diseases, malaria, typhoid, tuberculosis and chest infections

were treated through the mobile clinics and proper medication, supervised by the VHW. Patients suffering from serious diseases were brought to the hospital for investigation and treatment.

2. *Nutritional diseases:* Diseases caused by nutritional deficiencies such as anaemia, night blindness (erophthalmia), iodine deficiency (goitre) and rickets (calcium deficiency) were identified by the village-level worker, and referred to the hospital for investigation, diagnosis and treatment. Continuation of treatment was supervised by the VHW.

3. *Accidents:* VHWs learnt how to give first aid in an emergency and then referred patients for appropriate treatment.

4. *Maternal and child health, and family planning:* Rural women often do not have the health reserves required to bear the physiological strain of having a baby. Haemorrhage, sepsis, pre-eclamptic toxaemia of pregnancy, obstructed labour and abortion are killers of women. Underlying anaemia compounds these problems and leads to morbidity. Hence, it is important to recognize the factors that lead to these problems early. Arpana set up a system of checks and referrals to identify and manage such problems.

Arpana hospital has 75 beds and five disciplines: Medicine, Surgery, Obstetrics and Gynaecology, Ophthalmology and Dentistry

Maternal health

Pregnancy

1. *Identification of anaemia:* Home visits were made by the VHWs and TBAs from the third or fourth month of pregnancy. Cases of anaemia were recorded: the patient was given special care and iron and folic acid supplements. They also referred the pregnant woman to the mobile clinic for a check-up by the doctor. Haemoglobin was estimated at least twice during pregnancy. Thus, anaemic women were identified, treated and advised about their diets. Very severe cases were referred to the hospital.

2. *Iron, folic acid and calcium supplements* were distributed by health workers and TBAs to pregnant women for at least three months.

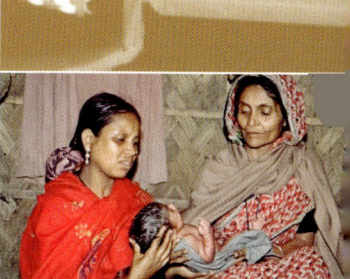

Paradigm shift through development programmes in selected villages of Haryana: Arpana Research and Charities Trust–India: 1993 (India)

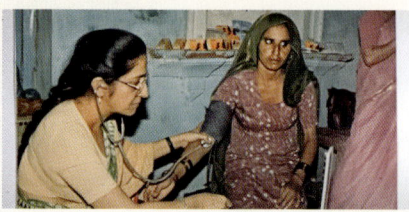
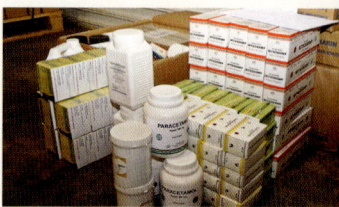

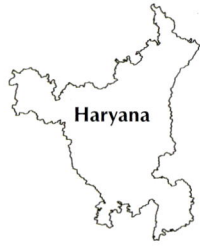
Haryana

Through home visits and discussions in cluster meetings, women were made aware of important health principles to follow during pregnancy and childbirth

3. *Immunization with tetanus toxoid:* motivated by the village workers, pregnant women took the scheduled injections of tetanus toxoid.

4. *Identification of pre-eclamptic toxaemia of pregnancy:* All village workers and TBAs were taught to recognize the signs and symptoms of this condition.

5. *Identification of high-risk mothers:* A special record was maintained of first-time pregnancies, especially among women below 18 or above 35 years of age; those in their fifth pregnancy or more; and those with a history of a previous difficult delivery, fetal loss or miscarriage. Abnormal positions and twin pregnancies were picked up by TBAs or at the antenatal clinics. TBAs were cautioned about these patients and taught how to recognize the danger signs so that they could refer them to the hospital in time.

6. *Health education:* Through home visits and discussions in cluster meetings, women were made aware of important health principles to follow during pregnancy and childbirth.

Childbirth or the natal period

1. *Clean methods of childbirth/prevention of sepsis:* TBAs were trained to use clean methods and were given midwifery kits. Each pregnant woman and her family was taught how to prepare a clean room, clean clothes, etc. for delivery.

2. *Haemorrhage:* High-risk cases were carefully watched for haemorrhage. TBAs dispensed tablets to help to control cases of haemorrhage after childbirth. They were taught to massage the uterus if severe haemorrhage occurred and make swift arrangements for referral if these measures did not elicit a response.

3. *Obstructed labour:* Early signs of obstructed labour, especially in high-risk pregnancies, were referred to the hospital to reduce the incidence of stillbirth and neonatal death.

Sasakawa Health Prize:
STORIES FROM SOUTH-EAST ASIA

Postnatal (postpartum) period

TBAs paid daily visits to the women they had delivered for 10 days and VHWs visited at least once a week. During this time they performed the following tasks: weighed the baby at birth; encouraged and promoted early breast-feeding including the nutrient-rich colostrums; identified haemorrhage and referred for treatment; identified and referred women with fever and sepsis; identified anaemic women for treatment; and advised mothers on breast-feeding. They also took care of the baby's cord, kept a record of the baby's weight, and washed and bathed the child and mother.

Child health

Growth monitoring: Growth monitoring began at birth. VHWs were provided weighing devices. If a baby's weight was normal, it was weighed once a month during the first year. Growth charts were given to the mother, and the purpose of the charts was explained. Initially, the mothers often used the charts to start fires. Later, the mothers valued the charts and looked after them carefully. VHWs recorded the baby's weight and other information about the child in a register. Malnourished children were identified and monitored carefully.

> Mothers were introduced to the concept of weaning foods, which gradually found acceptance, especially in those villages with a supplementary nutrition programme for children below six years of age

Nutrition: Mothers were introduced to the concept of weaning foods, which gradually found acceptance, especially in those villages with a supplementary nutrition programme for children below six years of age. The community contributed wheat and rice at each of the two major harvests, while Arpana contributed milk, vegetables, pulses, etc. for wholesome mid-day meals. Malnourished children and infants below one year of age were given a soft meal. This proved to be a strong argument against the prevalent belief that weaning foods could not be digested by children under one year of age – a belief which resulted in deficiencies and malnourishment of infants.

Day-care centres for preschool children: Children below six years of age were extremely vulnerable, as many working parents had to abandon them to the care of aged grandparents or young brothers and sisters. With no regular attention, they suffered from deficient and irregular meals and were unable to

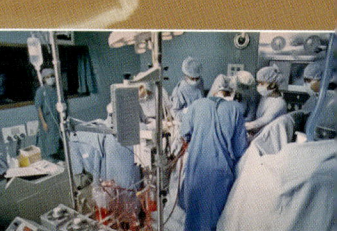

Children at Arpana day-care centres were provided with a warm, stimulating environment where they practised personal hygiene daily and learnt its importance

Paradigm shift through development programmes in selected villages of Haryana: Arpana Research and Charities Trust–India: 1993 (India)

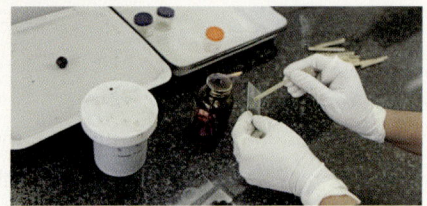 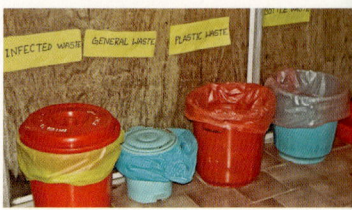

Haryana

Arpana trained village women to look after infants, with special attention to their cleanliness

acquire habits of personal hygiene. Children at Arpana day-care centres were provided with a warm, stimulating environment where they practised personal hygiene daily and learnt its importance; they participated in activities which encouraged the development of their motor and cognitive skills; learnt letters and numbers; practised clay modelling and simple creative activities; and participated in cooperative work and play. The children developed school going habits that helped them adjust to school later on. They were able to learn easily and quickly, and responded far better than other children. The drop-out rate decreased in this group of primary schoolchildren.

Creches: Arpana initially faced a great deal of mistrust in the rural community. This prevented mothers from leaving their preschool children in Arpana's care. This attitude changed over the years as the children's changed habits proved the efficacy of the preschool methods. Soon, large numbers of Arpana preschool centres had to respond to the demand of mothers to look after their infants.

Arpana trained village women to look after infants, with special attention to their cleanliness. A soft meal was added for infants below two-and-a-half years of age. Simple play activities stimulated their motor faculties, coordination and cognitive skills.

Immunization: Immunization was carried out against six major diseases and 85% of children below one year were completely immunized by 1992. Booster doses were given, followed by diphtheria–tetanus (DT) and tetanus toxoid (TT) immunizations for older children up to the age of 15 years. This was possible because mothers in Arpana's villages became aware, through street meetings and discussions with Arpana workers, of the need to immunize their children.

Vitamin A: Vitamin A supplements were given every six months to children until they were five years old as a prophylactic against blindness.

Other illnesses in children: The major killers of infants and small children were diarrhoea and pneumonia. All Arpana's village workers were given oral rehydration solution (ORS) and became adept at recognizing both dehydration and the danger signs of pneumonia in children.

Trained TBAs: TBAs were trained to encourage the village women to accept new methods of childrearing, healthy infant-feeding practices, preventive child health care, etc. This brought about a dramatic improvement in the health of rural mothers and their babies.

Family planning

Arpana instituted several programmes to improve the health of mothers and advise them on the need for family planning. The overall thrust of Arpana's programmes was to bring about a radical change in the status of women, without which family planning efforts would not have been effective. TBAs and female community health workers advised mothers with only one or two children to use temporary methods of family planning such as the copper-T and the pill. For those with two or more children, they advised tubectomy. The success of Arpana's family planning programme was possible only because of the infrastructure of health-care facilities that had been painstakingly built up, and its trained health workers. This brought about a profound change in the attitudes of the rural folk in the target villages. It took many years of hard work to inculcate a positive attitude, from the initial deep distrust of family planning. The contraceptive measures and sterilizations performed in Arpana's family planning programme reflected the success in changing attitudes towards the overall health-care programme at the grass-roots level.

Arpana's endeavours in family planning, in coordination with those of the State Government and the Chief Medical Officer, Karnal, contributed to the national effort in this critical area.

Arpana's health workers and helpers were responsible for recording information, i.e. the number of couples between 15 and 45 years, the number of children per couple, immunization, antenatal and postnatal care, babies' weight, etc. They also motivated couples for family planning through TBAs who had performed deliveries and given health care to babies. They supplied condoms and the pill to couples, as well as advice on family spacing. Education in health care and prevention was conducted from house to house and at village meetings. VHWs scripted a play on family planning and used traditional folk

> Mothers in Arpana's villages became aware, through street meetings and discussions with Arpana workers, of the need to immunize their children

> Arpana's endeavours in family planning, in coordination with those of the State Government and the Chief Medical Officer, Karnal, contributed to the national effort in this critical area

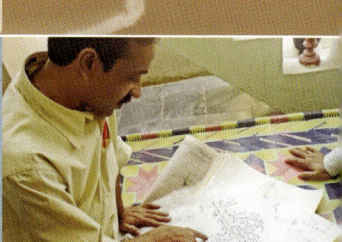

Paradigm shift through development programmes in selected villages of Haryana: Arpana Research and Charities Trust–India: 1993 (India)

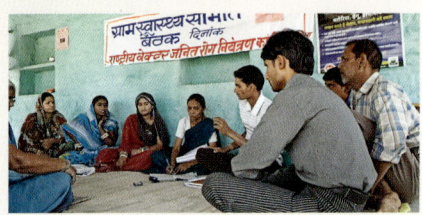
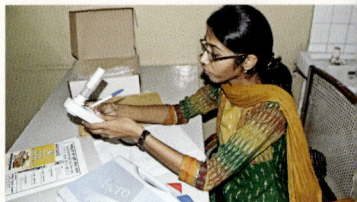

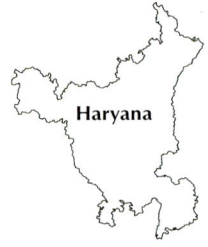

Haryana

> Arpana cooperated closely with the government, which supplied contraceptive devices as well as a small incentive for sterilization cases

songs to convey messages to rural audiences. Cases were referred to the mobile village clinic for fitting of copper-T, and to Arpana hospital for tubectomy or vasectomy operations.

From 1987 to 1991, 2436 operations were performed of cases referred from the primary and secondary levels. Transport for tubectomy patients was provided back to the patient's village. VHWs followed up on a house-to-house basis.

Arpana cooperated closely with the government, which supplied contraceptive devices as well as a small incentive for sterilization cases. Where there was a village government worker, by prior arrangement, Arpana provided health care and immunization, leaving family planning to the worker. Arpana received recognition as the best nongovernment organization (NGO) doing family planning work from the Haryana State Government for three years running. Encouragingly, the Block Development Officer began referring cases to Arpana hospital.

Health education

Health workers were trained to motivate families to space their children. Late marriage of girls was encouraged, as was a delay in the birth of the first child for newly married women. In Arpana's family planning effort, much importance was given to the education of women as well as to a reduction in neonatal and natal mortality.

Family planning camps

Arpana started a series of family planning camps at Arpana hospital, with teams of doctors from Delhi hospitals such as the All India Institute of Medical Sciences, Moolchand Hospital, Lady Hardinge Medical College, and Guru Tegh Bahadur Medical College. Laparascopic tubectomies were carried out at these camps.

5.3 Eye care

The objective of Arpana's large rural eye relief wing was to totally eliminate preventable blindness from an ever-widening target area by identifying those in need of operations at clinics and screening camps. Arpana brought them to the hospital for operations, provided aftercare, spectacles, food, etc. and then took them back to their villages.

In 1991, 2784 operations were performed at the hospital. Glaucoma and trachoma were also tackled, both through a preventive programme, and by hospital treatment where necessary. All facilities including food were provided free to eye patients referred from the rural camps, which especially benefited malnourished elderly patients living below the poverty line.

6. Conclusion and lessons learned

Arpana's programmes began in 1980 in 36 illiterate, economically disadvantaged villages of Haryana. The primary activity of Arpana's health programmes was awareness creation. With traditional, feudal mindsets, ignorance about germs and modern medicine, and old habits ingrained in all the communities, awareness needed to be generated for changes to be effected. This was carried out through VHWs who held street meetings in different neighbourhoods.

One of the most important lessons that emerged from Arpana's village-level health programmes was that rapport between VHWs and beneficiaries is vital to the success of such a programme. Arpana selected one or two promising villagers from each of the villages and trained them as village health and development workers. Once these workers were convinced of basic health principles and the actions necessary to implement them, they could in turn convince their fellow villagers. Capacity building and communication skills were built up along with basic health information and preventive interventions. VHWs provided information, guidance and counselling on a personal level to individuals and families. As the usefulness of their advice was proven over the years, their status grew in their families, communities and villages.

> All facilities including food were provided free to eye patients referred from the rural camps, which especially benefited malnourished elderly patients living below the poverty line

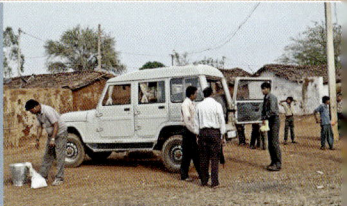

> Capacity building and communication skills were built up along with basic health information and preventive interventions. VHWs provided information, guidance and counselling on a personal level to individuals and families

PARADIGM SHIFT THROUGH DEVELOPMENT PROGRAMMES IN SELECTED VILLAGES OF HARYANA: ARPANA RESEARCH AND CHARITIES TRUST—INDIA: 1993 (INDIA)

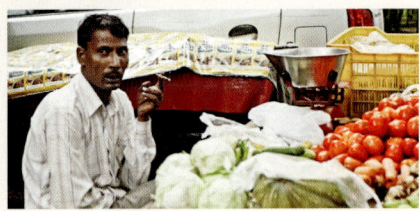 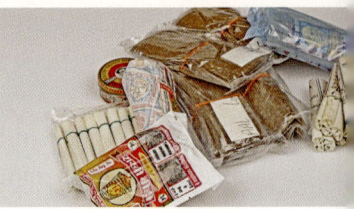

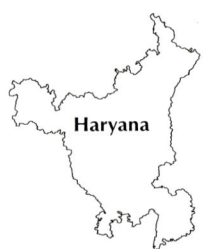

> Most family women such as the mother-in-law and sister-in-law did not know what a pregnant woman required. Even when informed, the family did not consider it necessary to send a pregnant woman for check-ups, immunization and supplements

TBAs were also sought out by Arpana and given special training in midwifery, including hygiene and cleanliness, recognizing high-risk pregnancies and record-keeping. Continual training was provided over the years aimed at overcoming their old habits and practices, especially their mindsets, on the unimportance of their jobs and the triviality of their inputs. TBAs gave feedback to Arpana in these sessions, which allowed changes to be made for greater effectiveness.

Arpana encouraged close cooperation between the VHWs and TBAs for the overall benefit of the villagers. Both their roles were given importance and they were encouraged to support each other. Both became links to the community, through the mobile clinics which came to their villages and to Arpana hospital, where they were recognized by the hospital staff and were able to get easy admittance/services for their patients. This helped them earn more respect from the village communities.

Arpana's programme was multifaceted and intensive. Pregnant women received information, guidance and support from VHWs and TBAs, along with check-ups, nutrition and supplements, as well as help with explaining the importance of antenatal care to their mothers-in-law. Most family women such as the mother-in-law and sister-in-law did not know what a pregnant woman required. Even when informed, the family did not consider it necessary to send a pregnant woman for check-ups, immunization and supplements. Thus, infant mortality rates and women's morbidity and mortality rates were high. VHWs and TBAs stressed the importance of check-ups, good diets, supplements and immunizations. They also brought the women to the monthly mobile clinics. They carefully recorded those at high risk, preparing them to go to the hospital for delivery. They spent hours counselling family members, especially the mother-in-law, about the necessity of antenatal care in order to have a healthy child. Marriage after 18 years of age, spacing and limiting the number of children through family planning were stressed, especially since 70% of the village women were anaemic and overworked.

Sasakawa Health Prize:
STORIES FROM SOUTH-EAST ASIA

Preschool children received day care in a loving ambience, and were taught through poems, stories and games. They also received nursery school education and learnt social cooperation.

Mothers participated in the mid-day meal both through donations of grain and through cooking nutritious and tasty meals.

Child health guides were schoolchildren who had attended the day-care centres. They were then trained in imparting basic health principles through skits, demonstrations of ORS (for diarrhoea), songs and rallies to build up preventive health activities in their own villages. They also participated in sanitation and cleanliness drives in their villages. Adolescent girls were involved in literacy programmes.

One of the most important aspects of Arpana's programmes was its record-keeping, monitoring and reporting. These were essential activities for gleaning information required for checking the efficacy of inputs. Programme changes were made from the information gathered meticulously on a monthly basis. This was a dynamic programme which responded to the local needs and effected changes from within.

> One of the most important aspects of Arpana's programmes was its record keeping, monitoring and reporting

The changes that Arpana sought from the community were not expensive. Kitchen gardens were encouraged through discussions, information, demonstrations and packets of seeds. VHWs helped women choose small plots of land, usually just outside their kitchens, for intensive cultivation of green leafy vegetables. Courtyards and small pockets of unused land were also found. Drainage water from hand pumps was used to irrigate gardens. Over 4000 kitchen gardens were planted and tended for years, providing essential nutrients to the anaemic women and girls of the villages.

Recognizing diarrhoea as a major killer of children five years old and below (WHO estimates that 25% of India's children in that age bracket die as a result of diarrhoea) resulted in an important initiative for diarrhoea management – home-made ORS.

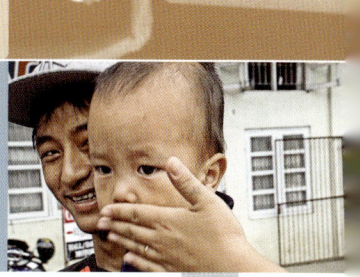

Preschool children received day care in a loving ambience, and were taught through poems, stories and games. They also received nursery school education and learnt social cooperation

PARADIGM SHIFT THROUGH
DEVELOPMENT PROGRAMMES
IN SELECTED VILLAGES OF
HARYANA: ARPANA RESEARCH
AND CHARITIES TRUST—INDIA:
1993 (INDIA)

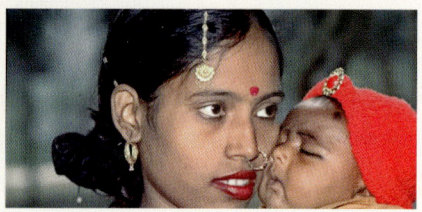
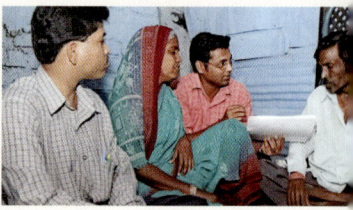

> The greatest weakness of the Arpana programme was its inability to have successful programmes for men

Improvement in sanitation and hygiene were also among the changes Arpana effected in the target villages. These included "clean courtyards" with food kept in ventilated cupboards screened against flies and insects, clean drinking water in covered earthen pots and accessed by clean cups, and private latrines kept hygienically clean.

Thus, Arpana's programmes effectively targeted the needs of the time, resulting in awareness creation and providing health care through a three-tier system of VHWs and TBAs, mobile clinics and a referral base hospital. As villagers became more aware, Arpana was able to move from being a provider of health services to an enabler. Women were empowered through Arpana-facilitated self-help groups (SHGs) in savings, micro-loans, entrepreneurship, civic governance and leadership. Arpana also motivated SHGs to take up health responsibilities of the community. Now SHGs are forming their own federations for a platform from which they can be a more effective source of support for their member groups in monetary resources, information sharing about government programmes, and liaising with officials and agencies.

Perhaps the greatest weakness of the Arpana programme was its inability to have successful programmes for men. These programmes were started, but it was soon realized that different types of inputs would be required. The male health workers required higher salaries/incentives. Different trainings were needed and different programmes required. Due to lack of funding, these programmes were not carried out.

7. Afterword

At the time of the Sasakawa candidature, Arpana's programmes basically provided health services and education not available to the beneficiaries by other means. This was the need of the time and Arpana did its utmost to provide these services.

However, as the government started providing more health coverage in villages, it was clear that the need for the disadvantaged was self-sufficiency in village health and greater economic security.

Sasakawa Health Prize:
STORIES FROM SOUTH-EAST ASIA

Thus, using the Sasakawa prize money and other resources, Arpana began a highly successful programme of women's SHGs. For greater economic security, training was given in entrepreneurship, record-keeping, accounts, communication, leadership, local governance, legal literacy, etc.

Today, there are 373 SHGs with 5004 members; 963 members have taken business loans and set up their own businesses. Now, not only do women have more economic resources, but their status has risen in the family and community as they are able to access loans and speak out on village issues at local council meetings.

Arpana development workers also trained women on basic health principles, which they share with their neighbours. They are motivated to take up health responsibilities in their neighbourhoods and are now looking after each pregnant woman, seeing that she receives at least three medical check-ups as well as the necessary immunizations and supplements. They check that neighbourhood children do not get malnourished and make sure that they receive all their immunizations. In addition, they inform their neighbours about the health services available to them through new government programmes. In short, they are developing self-sufficiency in health in their villages.

Arpana has facilitated two federations of 167 SHGs for women. These federations are platforms from which women's voices are heard and, increasingly, listened to with respect. They provide larger resources for loans, more information on government schemes for the poor, forums for discussion and plans of action. The women leaders have visited district and block officers on their own and their grievances have been heard and redressed. They work together to collectively present matters for action in village councils. They are enquiring into funds and schemes received by the councils and making their village councils transparent. Arpana salutes these women, and is deeply grateful for the encouragement and support rendered by the World Health Organization through the Sasakawa Health Prize.

> Arpana development workers are motivated to take up health responsibilities in their neighbourhoods and are now looking after each pregnant woman, seeing that she receives at least three medical check-ups as well as the necessary immunizations and supplements

> The women leaders have visited district and block officers on their own and their grievances have been heard and redressed. They work together to collectively present matters for action in village councils

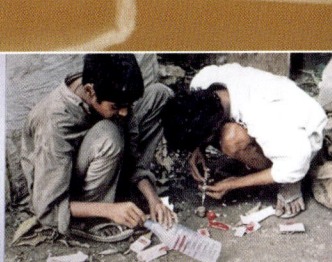

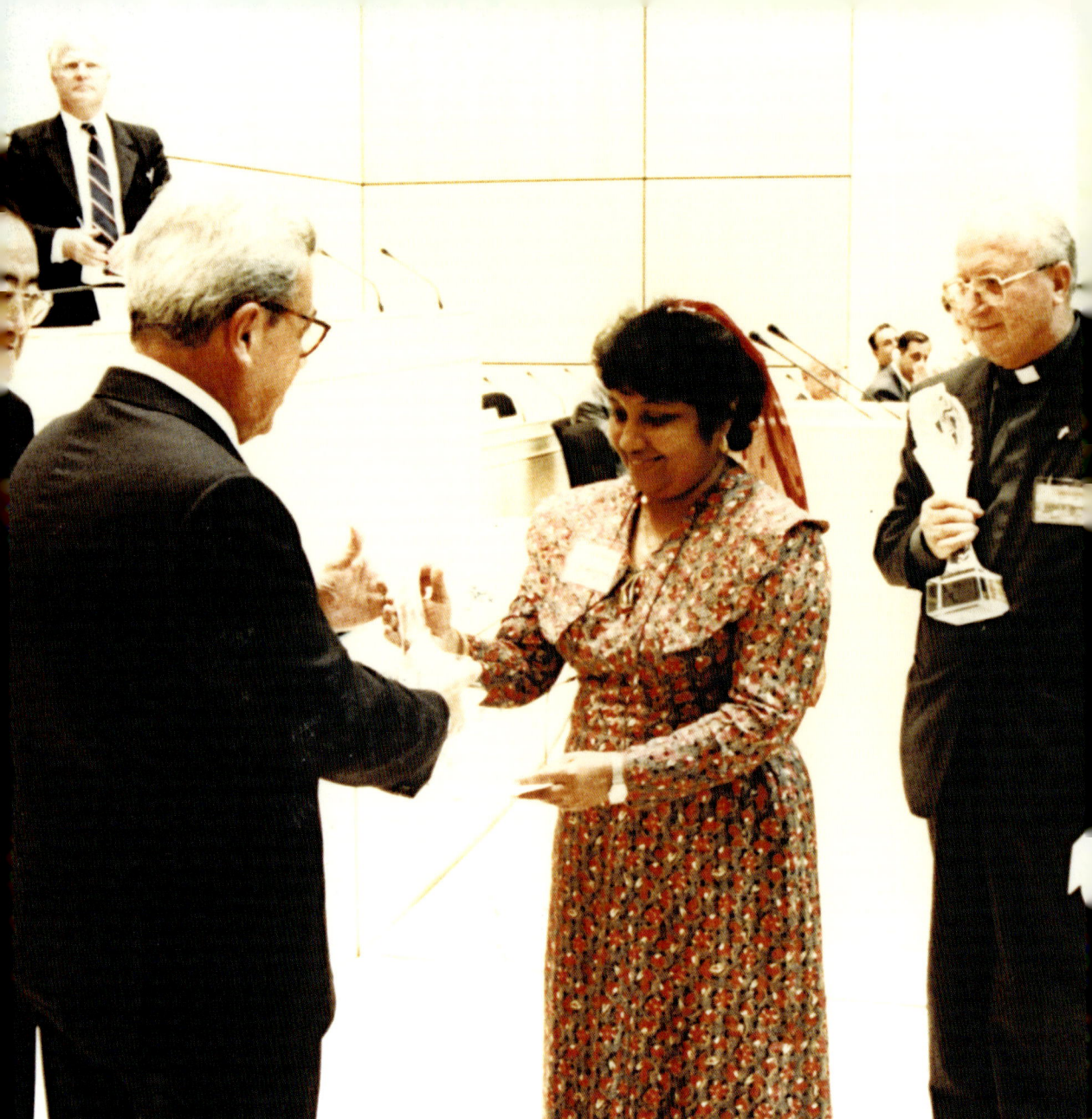

Dr Naila Firdous, representative of the Society for Health Education receives the 1996 Sasakawa Health Prize from the President of the 49th World Health Assembly.

WHO Photo

CHAPTER 8

1996

Society for Health Education (SHE): Maldives[*]

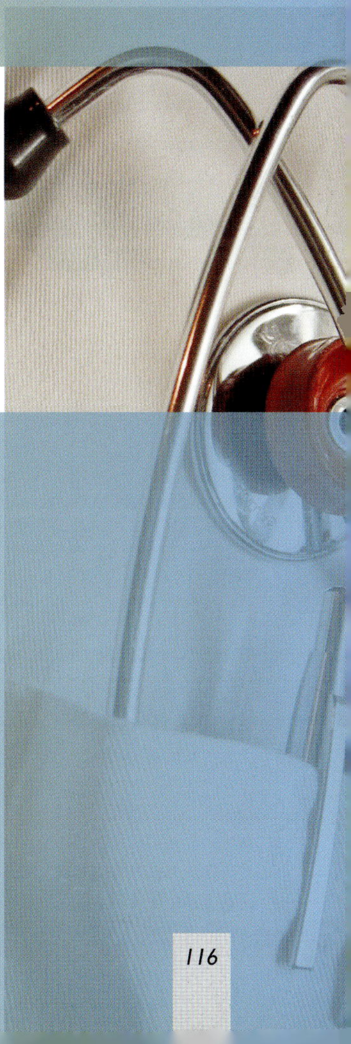

Recipient:
Society for Health Education
(Maldives)

[*] Draft prepared by Mrs Asna Luthfee
Programme Associate, Society for Health Education, Male, Maldives

The Society for Health Education (SHE) was established in 1988 with the objective of raising awareness on health and social issues among the people of the Maldives

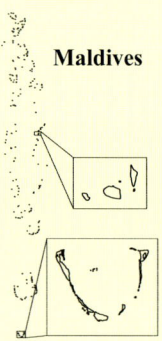

Maldives

The organization aims to foster family well-being in general and empower families and women in particular to make informed choices when seeking services from medical professionals

1. Introduction

The Society for Health Education (SHE) was established in 1988 with the objective of raising awareness on health and social issues among the people of the Maldives. The organization aims to foster family well-being in general and empower families and women in particular to make informed choices when seeking services from medical professionals. Awareness-raising by the organization comprises a wide range of activities, including publication and dissemination of print materials, conducting radio programmes and organization of public forums. At the time of establishment of the organization, health facilities were lacking in the majority of island communities. SHE's awareness-raising activities became popular among disadvantaged and remote island communities. These interactions contributed to the launching of parallel programmes on family planning, psychosocial counselling and thalassemia prevention. At the central level, in Male', the organization operates a family planning clinic, a counselling unit and a laboratory specialized in thalassemia screening.

Since its inception in 1988, SHE continues to explore options and the means to enhance the quality of life of Maldivian families. The organization reaffirms its commitment to sustaining these initiatives, and to further increasing public awareness on issues that influence family well-being. Effectiveness of health promotion initiatives are ensured by adopting suitable service delivery mechanisms, fostering improvements in reproductive health parameters, continuing thalassemia-prevention activities, promoting responsible parenthood concepts, facilitating empowerment of women and youth, supporting victims of abuse, extending counselling to adolescents and families, and encouraging community ownership of development.

1.1 Specific goals

1. Increase public awareness on the implications and consequences of crucial social and health concerns including large family size, high divorce rate, smoking habits, spread of drug use, large proportion of adolescents and youth.

2. Promote marital stability by improving the reproductive health status of women, popularizing responsible parenthood concepts and strengthening related services.

3. Minimize the detrimental effects of marital instability, divorce, abuse, and other habits and practices that affect family well-being.

2. Programme description

2.1 Counselling and psychosocial support services

During the past 18 years, SHE has introduced a number of services to Maldivian society. Among them, counselling has gained popular acceptance and has been formally integrated into social services and education establishments. When SHE introduced counselling support services in 1988, nuisance calls to its helpline were not uncommon. This service is now popularly recognized as one of the most dependable and credible counselling services in the country.

Counselling support services comprise face-to-face counselling, a telephone helpline and play therapy for young children. Currently, counselling services are provided for around 500 clients annually. There is a significant unmet need for counselling, which has been confirmed by a number of assessments and interactions with the community. However, the country's unique geography and developing public administration system are not conducive to the expansion of this service. In particular, public perception of services provided by nongovernmental organizations (NGOs) as intermediary interventions remains a challenge that needs to be addressed effectively.

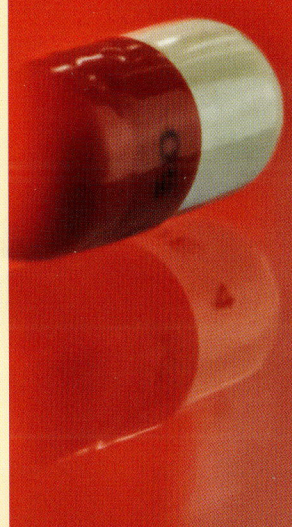

SHE's awareness raising activities became popular among disadvantaged and remote island communities

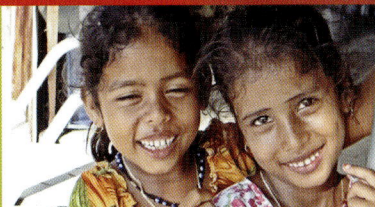

Since its inception in 1988, SHE continues to explore options and the means to enhance the quality of life of Maldivian families

SOCIETY FOR HEALTH EDUCATION (SHE):
MALDIVES: 1996 (MALDIVES)

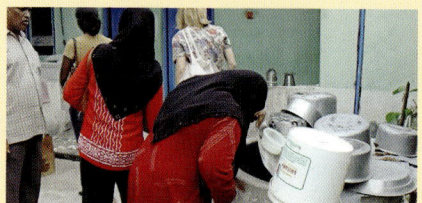
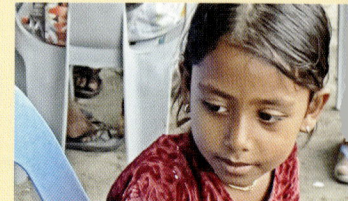

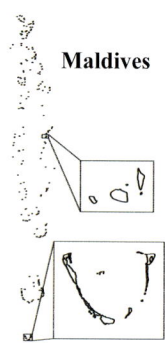
Maldives

Family planning was rightly accorded high priority by the Society during the early years. Raising awareness on family planning was a key component of the health promotion activities of the Society

2.2 Family planning

The Maldives experienced a population boom during the 1970s and 1980s, created by a fast-declining mortality rate and continuing high fertility levels. Even by the early 1980s, the growth rate of the Maldivian population remained above 3% and the total fertility rate (TFR) exceeded the six children level.

Family planning was rightly accorded high priority by the Society during the early years. Raising awareness on family planning was a key component of the health promotion activities of the Society. The issue was addressed through print materials and public forums. Eventually, with the support of the United Nations Population Fund (UNFPA) and the International Planned Parenthood Federation (IPPF), SHE established the first clinic for family planning in the Maldives called the Family Planning Clinic (FPC). It remains the only clinic in the Maldives providing family planning services outside the government structure.

FPC currently serves more than 1300 regular customers. Services include provision of pills, condoms, injectable contraceptives and intrauterine devices (IUDs). Though the clinic targets an annual service output of 600 couple-year protection rate (CYPR), it manages to achieve a CYPR of around 400.

FPC is being transformed into a centre providing ancillary services related to family planning and aims to eventually introduce most components of the reproductive health framework. Establishment of an awareness-raising service on youth, and for youth, under the banner of "Youth Kiosk" was a significant development. In the Maldives, the youth comprise more than 25% of the population and youth-related issues pose serious challenges to development planning. The Youth Kiosk provides special awareness-raising sessions for youth visiting the premises, particularly for those visiting for thalassaemia screening. These sessions provide pre-marriage counselling and information on sexual health and responsible parenthood. Around 1000 youth seek the support of the kiosk annually.

2.3 Health promotion

The themes addressed under this programme cover a wide range of issues such as family planning, nutrition, drug use, personal hygiene, thalassaemia and other genetically inherited diseases, pregnancy and responsible parenthood, environmental health and prevention of smoking.

Health promotion activities aim to provide access to beneficiaries with minimum inconvenience through various modalities. However, the effectiveness of some of the modalities gradually loses relevance with developmental progress. For example, print materials have become less effective with the expansion of radio and television. Public forums also have become less convenient with changing lifestyles and competing commitments. The Society endeavours to sustain its health promotion activities even in a restrictive setting.

Under this programme, the Society publishes a monthly leaflet (Kulunu) and broadcasts a weekly radio programme. A wide range of topics have already been addressed through these outlets, ranging from personal hygiene to alpha-thalassaemia. Two modalities were used to extend selected services to the periphery. Initially, a mobile health team (designated as multipurpose health trip – MPHT) was fielded to targeted localities. The purpose of the field visit was to organize awareness-raising activities at the community level and extend selected medical services. The team comprised medical doctors, nurses, counsellors and health educators. The combined provision of medical services and awareness-raising activities helped to attract more people to the various programmes organized on these trips.

MPHT was highly relevant to those communities where there is no health service outlet. However, with the increasing number of health posts in the Atoll region, the relevance of the mobile team has diminished gradually. The effectiveness of these visits was sustained by increasing the number of specialists joining the team.

Another modality introduced under the health promotion programme is the organization of a community festival (Health Festival) to address continuing and emerging issues such as reproductive health, food and nutrition, smoking, drug use and youth.

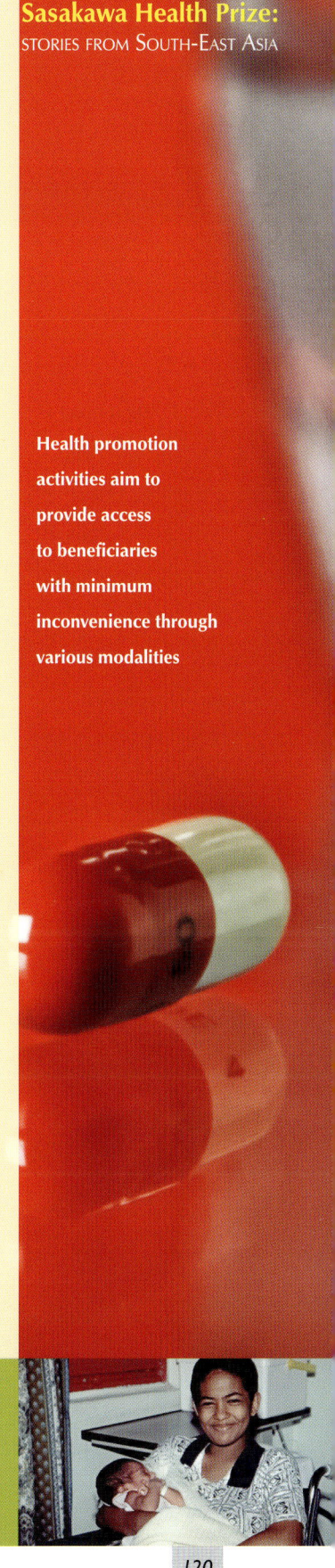

Sasakawa Health Prize: STORIES FROM SOUTH-EAST ASIA

> Health promotion activities aim to provide access to beneficiaries with minimum inconvenience through various modalities

> Public forums have become less convenient with changing lifestyles and competing commitments. The Society endeavours to sustain its health promotion activities even in a restrictive setting

Society for Health Education (SHE):
Maldives: 1996 (Maldives)

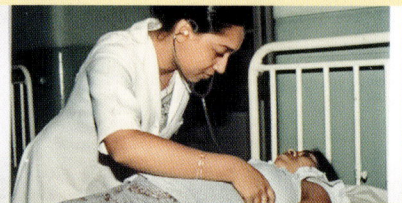 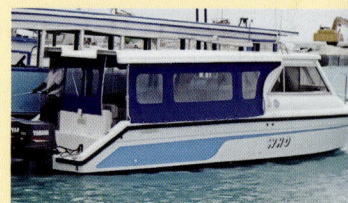

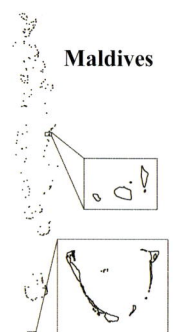
Maldives

Society organizes a special awareness-raising programme for students of secondary schools in Male. Under this programme, students of grades 9 and 10 are given an opportunity to clarify issues that concern them

The Society organizes a special awareness-raising programme for students of secondary schools in Male'. Under this programme, students of grades 9 and 10 are given an opportunity to clarify issues that concern them. These sessions are guided by resource people and create an open environment for students to raise sensitive issues about their personal and family life, schooling, reproductive health, and nutrition and career prospects.

2.4 Facilitating people-centred development

Population and family planning issues have remained a significant component of the health promotion activities of the Society. With a contraceptive prevalence rate of 32%, SHE's services are particularly required to desensitize family planning matters among both men and women in urban and rural areas.

SHE also focuses on addressing matters related to mental stress and related strains associated with a rapidly modernizing society. The Society remains prominent in this area because of its pioneering role in introducing and popularizing counselling as a viable treatment option. It provides telephone as well as face-to-face counselling.

SHE has created innovative programmes to achieve health promotion, including the organization of a series of health exhibitions, which has proved to be effective in changing attitudes and promoting health-conscious lifestyles. SHE has organized seven exhibitions in three atolls. These exhibitions addressed a wide range of topics and issues. In addition to setting up informative displays, the exhibition facilitated clarification of issues directly from relevant professionals drawn from the pool of experts available in the country.

SHE is actively involved in the promotion of other issues related to health and family such as reproductive health, healthy lifestyles, nutrition and dietary habits, empowerment of women, proper utilization of medical services and participatory development. Public awareness on these issues is raised through printed materials, public meetings, and radio and TV programmes. Along with awareness raising, SHE has also taken initiatives in developing infrastructure in the atolls. Under this initiative, four community centres have been constructed in two atolls.

3. Challenges

While socioeconomic development is progressing well, certain areas of the social sector demand urgent attention. Public awareness of specific health and social issues such as nutrition and healthy dietary habits, healthy lifestyles, contraceptive acceptance, attitudinal changes to achieve better health, and mental health and related issues are areas that need to be addressed. For example, improvements in the nutritional situation fall far short of those achieved in other health-related areas. Studies undertaken in 1990 by the government and the United Nations Children's Fund (UNICEF) reaffirmed that child nutrition is a problem that has to be addressed effectively. It was found that malnutrition persists at an unacceptably high rate; about one third of children had stunting, 17% had wasting and 44% were malnourished.

4. Winning the Sasakawa Health Prize

Since its inception until the time of the award, SHE was a pioneer in advancing the reach of primary health care to marginalized and geographically isolated populations of the country. At that time, the primary health care system in these communities was minimal, even though there were many health posts. However, ground-breaking modalities such as the MPHT led to a notable improvement in the quality of health care available in these geographically disadvantaged communities. Along with this, the creation of innovative programmes to address emerging health issues also contributed to the effective and efficient management of health systems and policy developments. For example, the health exhibitions held in the islands was something new at that time, as SHE's exhibitions differed from others, with live demonstrations such as showing how to prepare nutritious food.

Even though such exemplary work by SHE acted as the platform for recognition by the country's communities and the government (such as winning the most prestigious award in the country given by the President – Public Service Award for innovative work in health care), SHE's interaction with partners in the international arena was minimal. In order to broaden its horizon and form international alliances, the organization considered global recognition necessary

> SHE's services are particularly required to desensitize family planning matters among both men and women in urban and rural areas

> Since its inception until the time of the award, SHE was a pioneer in advancing the reach of primary health care to marginalized and geographically isolated populations of the country

SOCIETY FOR HEALTH EDUCATION (SHE):
MALDIVES: 1996 (MALDIVES)

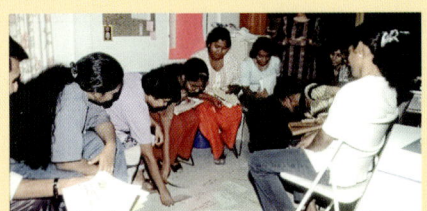 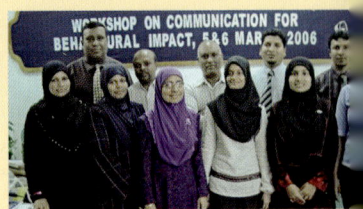

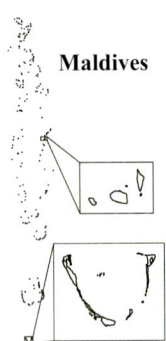
Maldives

SHE made use of information, education and communication (IEC) methods in enhancing the knowledge of the public, especially of marginalized communities

to further strengthen its work and overcome challenges. International recognition such as the Sasakawa Health Prize opened up numerous opportunities to sustain SHE's goal of providing innovative health care to the country.

5. Post-Sasakawa Health Prize

Since the Sasakawa Health Prize in 1996, the past 15 years have seen dramatic changes in the methods of service delivery by SHE. With the worldwide social, economic, political and cultural changes, SHE once again took initiatives in adopting contemporary methods that have proven to be highly effective for service delivery.

As mentioned earlier, SHE made use of information, education and communication (IEC) methods in enhancing the knowledge of the public, especially of marginalized communities. Though IEC leaflets and via radio broadcasts had been proven effective in the Maldives in the past, these methods became obsolete. As the demand for knowledge on specific health and social issues continued, the behavioural changes seen through IEC regarding such issues diminished. SHE has since then adopted behavioural change communication (BCC) methods. The BCC campaigns carried out by SHE made use of the current technology in the country including mass media campaigns for identified vulnerable groups. For example, the mass media campaign under the BCC component of HIV/AIDS Global Fund Programme ensured that certain messages were instilled to effectively change behavioural patterns with regard to safe sex practices.

With economic changes throughout the world, SHE experienced financial restrictions, which greatly limited the number of health camps/festivals in the atolls. SHE thus adopted another concept – educating peers. These peers were chosen from within geographically isolated communities and trained by service providers at SHE. This proved not only cost effective in the long run, but extremely beneficial as these peer educators had as much impact in delivering services and information to their own communities as the teams from SHE. One effective example is that of peer educators trained from among migrant workers, who provide HIV/AIDS information to their people.

Sasakawa Health Prize:
STORIES FROM SOUTH-EAST ASIA

The past 15 years also saw in-house services get stronger as more qualified and educated staff joined the in-house reproductive health clinic, laboratory and counselling unit. A number of staff were trained in the Maldives and abroad to broaden and develop services. With the help of these trained persons, a successful community centre was developed in V. Atoll, where the locals were trained to maintain the centre.

SHE also formed alliances with both global and local partners in order to generate funds to sustain services. With these partnerships in place, the organization took initiatives to introduce more focus areas into its mandate. SHE became a member of IPPF in 1999, introducing new components such as advocacy, unsafe abortion and AIDS to its mandate. Strategies to successfully advocate for amendment in the restrictive rules and policies on abortion for rape and incest victims have also been established through this programme and will be implemented in the near future.

A similar alliance was formed with the Global Fund to fight AIDS, Tuberculosis and Malaria (Global Fund) to combat HIV/AIDS in the country. The goal of this was to continue to maintain Maldives as a low HIV prevalence country through appropriate and curative interventions. This alliance recognizes the importance of creating a supportive environment, to ensure not only support for HIV/AIDS initiatives but also to reduce the stigma and discrimination that people with HIV/AIDS often face. The main areas of work for SHE is community outreach, and creating a preventive and supportive environment through BCC activities.

Local partnerships were also forged with the government, which led to the recent introduction of the voluntary counselling and testing centre for HIV/AIDS in the premises of SHE. Supported by the Centre for Community Health and Disease Control (CCHDC of the government) and by the Global Fund, SHE staff were trained to handle VCT clients. SHE continues to work with civil society and community-based organizations in the new areas included in its mandate. Some of these organizations include SWAD (Society for Women Against Drugs), JOURNEY, UNDP and UNFPA. SHE has many activities in its Annual Programme Budget for 2011, which will allow NGOs in the selected islands such as Gdh. Thinadhoo, Addu Atoll to be trained, so that they could act as sub-partners, delivering services on behalf of SHE in their own island communities.

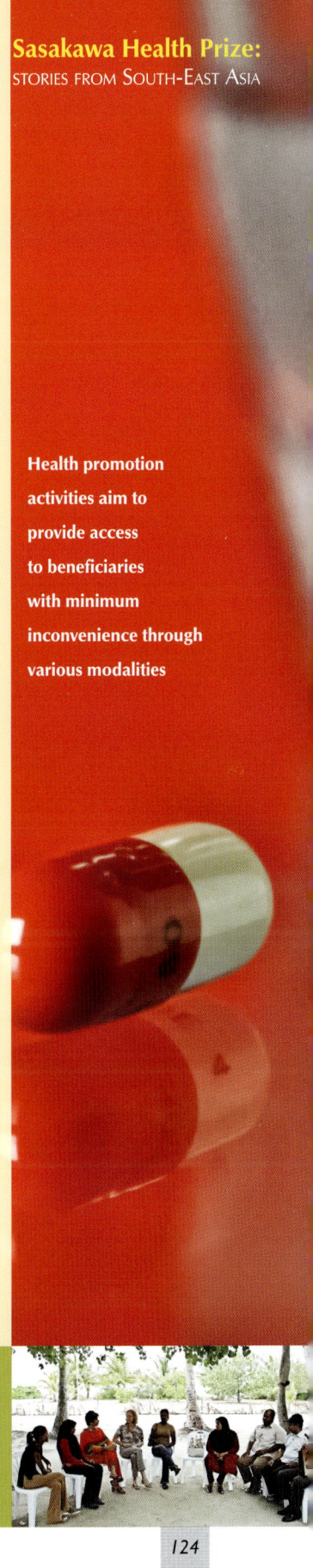

Health promotion activities aim to provide access to beneficiaries with minimum inconvenience through various modalities

> SHE continues to work with civil society and community-based organizations in the new areas included in its mandate. Some of these organizations include SWAD (Society for Women Against Drugs), JOURNEY, UNDP and UNFPA

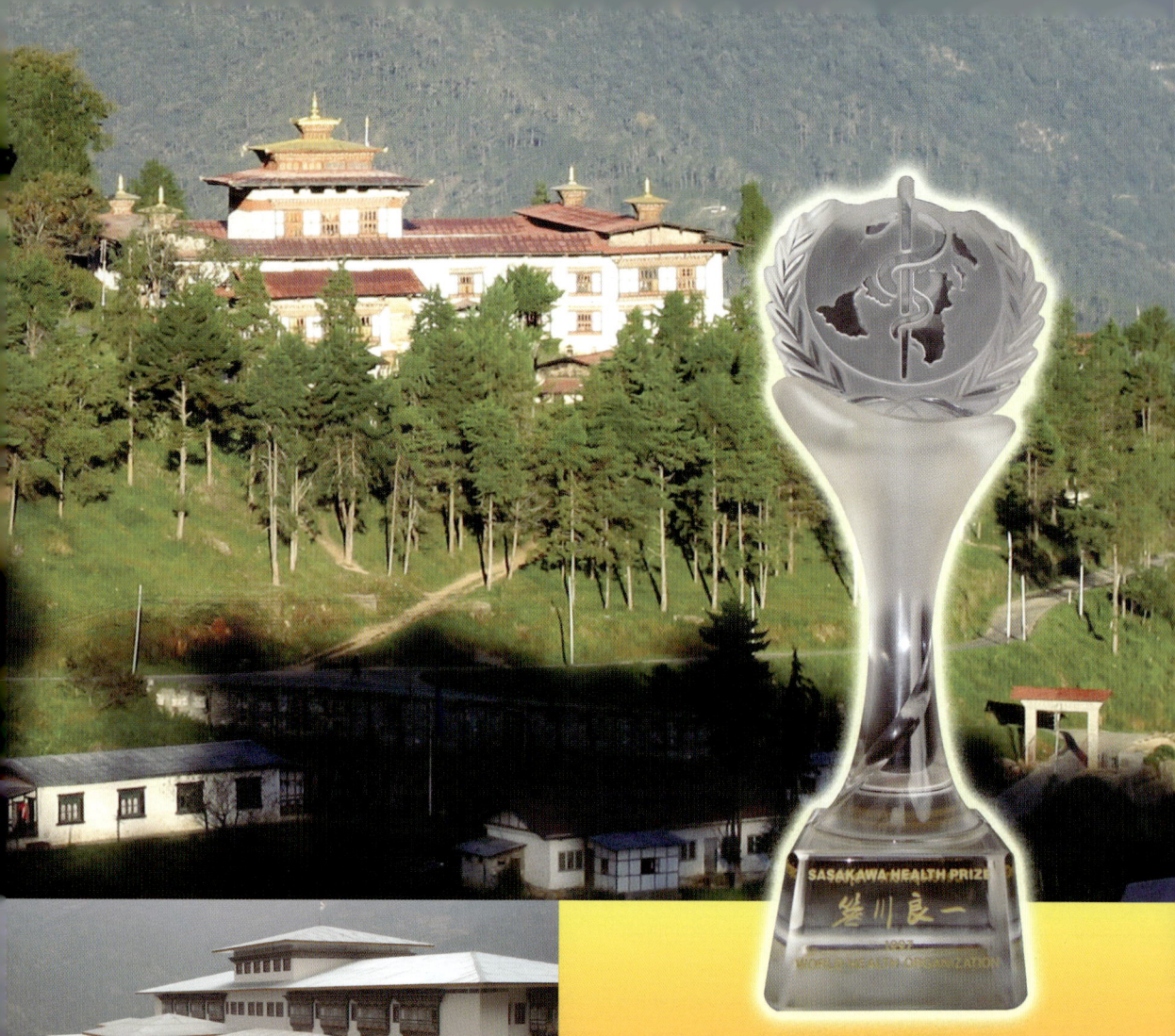

In recognition of the achievement in Health Development in Bhutan. Mongar Health Service Development Project won the WHO (SASAKAWA HEALTH PRIZE and AWARD) in 1997.

Mongar Health Services Development Project win the 1997 Sasakawa Health Prize at the World Health Assembly for innovative work in health services development.

Photo credit: Ministry of Health, Bhutan

CHAPTER 9

1997

Mongar health services development project: Bhutan[*]

Recipient:
The Mongar Health Services Development Project
(Bhutan)

[*] Draft prepared by Dr Sonam Ugen
Community Health Department,
Jigme Dorji Wangchuck National Referral Hospital (JDWNRH),
Ministry of Health, Royal Government of Bhutan

B hutan was awarded the prestigious Sasakawa Health Prize in 1997 for the success of the pilot project on primary health care implemented in Mongar Dzongkhag

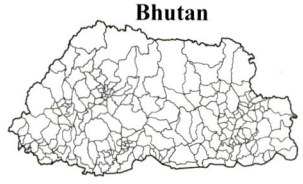

Bhutan

1. Introduction

The 1978 Alma-Ata international conference on primary health care set in motion collaboration and partnerships with rural communities in the Kingdom of Bhutan. The background for this move was the goal of the World Health Organization (WHO) to provide "Health for All" by the year 2000. For a country with rudimentary health infrastructure compounded with problems of accessibility, logistics, and lack of skilled human resources and funding, the global call then seemed a far cry. Within a few decades of planned development, the success of primary health care in Bhutan was proven beyond doubt. Bhutan's national health system now exemplifies an ideal model in primary health care. It is a well-thought out, well-planned system that actually works.

Within a few decades of planned development, the success of primary health care in Bhutan was proven beyond doubt

Bhutan was awarded the prestigious Sasakawa Health Prize in 1997 for the success of the pilot project on primary health care implemented in Mongar Dzongkhag. Bhutan's success story shows how the experience of one district in the mountainous Kingdom of Bhutan could lead to nationwide success in primary health care through partnerships.

2. Bhutan health services – a historical perspective

The history of planned socioeconomic development dates back to 1961, the year Bhutan embarked on its First Five-Year Plan. Before this period, health services were delivered through rudimentary facilities by a couple of doctors and a few compounders.

The difficult terrain, rough climatic conditions, scattered population, shortage of skilled human resources and scarce internal resources posed serious challenges to health-care delivery in the country. These problems were further compounded by the people's perception of illness, which was deeply rooted in strong cultural beliefs and superstition. This situation prevailed in most parts of the country. For treatment, the common person looked mainly to spiritual and ritual remedies and, in many instances, sought modern health care only as a last resort.

Health indicators of Bhutan during this period were among the poorest in the world. Infant and child morbidity and mortality rates were very high and largely attributable to diarrhoeal diseases, respiratory tract and parasitic infections. The major communicable diseases affecting the population in the 1960s and 1970s were tuberculosis, leprosy, malaria and smallpox. The problems of goitre and trachoma were also highly prevalent in the country.

Specific data on the nutritional situation are not available and very little is known about the dietary habits of the people. However, available information suggests that malnutrition with considerable stunting was common, mostly due to poor nutrition and recurrent infections. The risk of malnutrition, especially a deficiency of micronutrients, was perceived to be high among pregnant women, lactating mothers and preschool children. Morbidity and mortality among these groups were especially high.

3.   Modern health services

The foundation of a modern health-care delivery system was laid during the First Five-Year Plan period (1961–1966). At that time, services were largely curative and provided through a rudimentary health infrastructure. Due to shortage of skilled human resources for health, Bhutan was highly dependent on doctors and other categories of health personnel from neighbouring India and abroad.

By the end of the Fourth Plan period (1976/77–1980/81), comprehensive primary health care services were offered across the country through 65 basic health units (BHUs) and 22 hospitals. The establishment of the Royal Institute for Health Sciences (RIHS, earlier known as the Health School) in 1974 set the country on the road to self-reliance in human resources for health. Various categories of multipurpose primary health care workers

Health indicators of Bhutan during were among the poorest in the world

The foundation of a modern health-care delivery system was laid during the First Five-Year Plan period (1961–1966). Services were largely curative and provided through a rudimentary health infrastructure

MONGAR HEALTH SERVICES
DEVELOPMENT PROJECT:
BHUTAN: 1997 (BHUTAN)

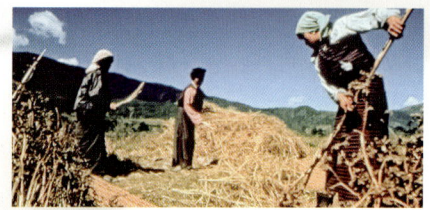
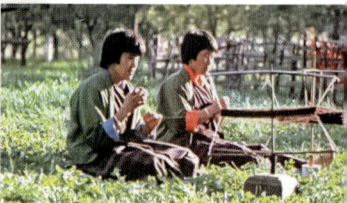
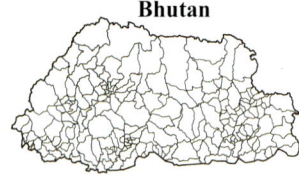

Bhutan

> The Royal Government established clearly defined national objectives related to health, which reflected the nation's commitment to primary health care

and nurses were trained at the RIHS. The National Health Policy aimed to provide free, integrated, equitable, cost-effective and well-balanced health services in the country.

This unprecedented progress within a span of two decades is attributed to visionary and strong leadership, a consistent national strategy and the generous support of bilateral and multilateral partners the Government of India (GOI), WHO, UNICEF, UNFPA, UNDP and DANIDA.

3.1 Commitment to primary health care

The actual thrust to modern health development came after the Alma-Ata Declaration on primary health care in 1978. In 1979, as a signatory to the Declaration, Bhutan adopted the primary health care strategy to achieve the social goal of Health for All by the year 2000. The Royal Government established clearly defined national objectives related to health, which reflected the nation's commitment to primary health care. During each successive Plan period, the health system was refined and streamlined to meet the essential elements of primary health care.

Bhutan's Fifth Five-Year Plan was geared to strengthen health infrastructure and expand coverage of essential health services. The Health Policy was aimed at attaining the highest level of health for the people of Bhutan through the primary health care approach. Accordingly, emphasis was shifted from mainly curative care to a mixture of curative, preventive, promotive and rehabilitative services. A system of integrated service delivery with a focus on expansion of the rural health services formed a component of the overall social development. The shift was aimed at eliminating disparities in health service delivery between different population groups and improving the situation in underprivileged and underserved areas.

The eight essential elements of primary health care included in the health-care package were:

- Health education
- Nutrition and food supply
- Water and sanitation
- Maternal and child welfare and family planning
- Immunization
- Control of communicable disease
- Treatment of common diseases, and
- Supply of essential drugs

These and other key areas were addressed through a series of programmes with the aim of strengthening general service delivery at all levels. The Royal Government also recognized the need to strengthen intersectoral collaboration, community participation, and improve referral from and support to peripheral health units.

4. District model health project

In pursuit of maximizing "Health for All by the year 2000" and community participation, a model health project was developed with WHO support. The explicit objective was to identify appropriate strategies, technologies and supporting systems, which were major areas of weakness in the primary health care system.

The model was based on several desirable features:

1. *Community involvement:* to ensure the participation of local people in their own health development by involving them at the formulation and operational phases.

2. *Intersectoral collaboration:* to garner support for the project from the district administration and other sectors during all phases.

3. *Sustainability:* to ensure that the health care delivery system would be capable of continuing steadily without critical dependence on external inputs.

4. *Cost-effectiveness:* the use of appropriate technology and locally available resources such as administrative set-up, human resources, construction material etc.

> The Royal Government also recognized the need to strengthen intersectoral collaboration, community participation, and improve referral from and support to peripheral health unit

> The Health Policy was aimed at attaining the highest level of health for the people of Bhutan through the primary health care approach

MONGAR HEALTH SERVICES DEVELOPMENT PROJECT:
BHUTAN: 1997 (BHUTAN)

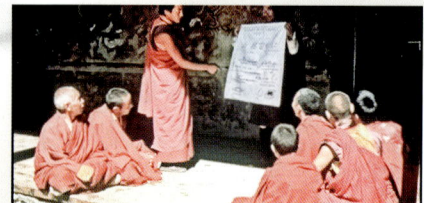 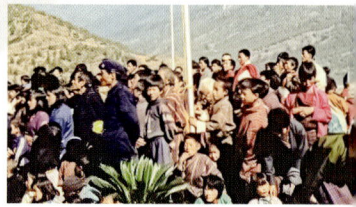

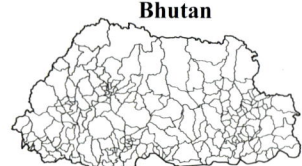
Bhutan

Health facilities in Mongar were grossly understaffed. An ambulance was seldom available to transport seriously ill patients

The district of Mongar was selected as the pilot area based on the premise that the district represented the country well in several medical and geophysical aspects. The health problems faced were typical of those in the eastern and central regions. The developmental constraints with respect to transport and communication applied to Mongar as well as other districts.

4.1 Overview of Mongar district

Mongar district is located in the eastern region of Bhutan and encompasses 1830 sq. km of rough and mountainous terrain with swift-flowing rivers.

In 1985, the population of Mongar District was estimated at 81 834. The whole district was divided into 11 gewogs (blocks) and each gewog in turn consisted of 20 chiwogs (village units). Houses were scattered on the slopes of mountains and most of the gewogs were located at a walking distance of 2–5 days from the district centre. The majority of the population are subsistence farmers who, apart from growing vegetables and fruits, also keep some livestock.

The district reported a literacy rate of 10%–20% Apart from seven primary schools and one high school, there were several religious learning centres, 10 agriculture extension centres and six animal husbandry centres distributed across the district.

Health facilities in Mongar at the start of the project comprised a District-cum-Leprosy Hospital, five BHUs and three dispensaries that catered to nearby villages. These facilities provided largely curative services with little or no involvement of the community.

Like other parts of the country, the health facilities in Mongar were grossly understaffed. An ambulance was seldom available to transport seriously ill patients.

4.2 Situational analysis

Health facilities in the district lacked reliable and uniform health information. Therefore, a survey was planned to develop baseline data for the Mongar district health project. The survey was conducted by teams of health workers in 10 randomly selected villages.

Sanitary conditions

No sanitary activity was initiated in the villages surveyed. It was observed that 90% of the surveyed population were defecating in the open fields. Some form of open latrine system was being used in some villages; others had poorly constructed pit latrines. The survey also revealed that most of the villages in Mongar reared pigs and cattle in the ground floor of houses or adjacent to them.

Water supply

Water supply schemes during the project period were under the jurisdiction of the District Public Works Division. Only a few of the houses in the villages surveyed had access to a piped water supply. For instance, only two out of the 52 houses in Ganglapong village received a water supply. The schemes were undertaken on individual request and not based on a needs assessment of the villages. Therefore, it was not surprising to note that several houses in a village remained without water supply. The survey also revealed that people often refrained from requesting for the scheme to avoid compulsory contribution of labour.

Though they were elements of health care, water supply and sanitation were implemented in isolation and not introduced with health education. The health sector was seldom involved in planning and implementing schemes in the rural areas.

Nutrition

Food consisted mainly of staple crops. Although most houses had a kitchen garden, the vegetables grown were limited to chillies, radish, potatoes and a few leafy vegetables. The incidence of anaemia and malnutrition was high in the villages surveyed. Women and children were largely affected.

Sasakawa Health Prize:
STORIES FROM SOUTH-EAST ASIA

> 90% of the surveyed population were defecating in the open fields. Some form of open latrine system was being used in some villages; others had poorly constructed pit latrines

> The health sector was seldom involved in planning and implementing schemes in the rural areas

Mongar health services development project:
Bhutan: 1997 (Bhutan)

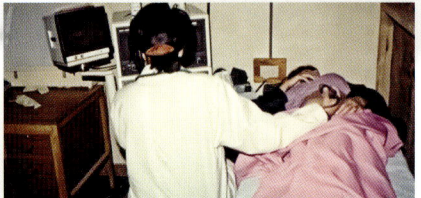
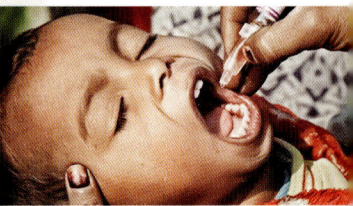

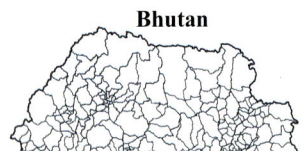

> It was observed that people were generally cooperative and fairly open to new ideas when approached with the right attitude

Health-seeking behaviour

Although predominantly a Buddhist society, the practice of rites and rituals was not uncommon and varied from village to village. In a few villages, black magic, poisoning and traditional healers hindered acceptance of health programmes. Cultural beliefs compounded by superstition prevented local communities from seeking help from the health facilities. It was observed that people were generally cooperative and fairly open to new ideas when approached with the right attitude.

Common disease and health indicators

District health data revealed that 80% of the illnesses were communicable in nature and directly or indirectly transmitted through human feces, largely attributed to poor sanitation and hygiene. The most common health problems reported were diarrhoea, dysentery, respiratory tract infections, worm infestations and skin diseases. Malnutrition was especially common among women and children. The important health indicators reported at the outset of the project were as follows:

- Crude death rate: 16/1000 population
- Crude birth rate: 28/1000 population
- Infant mortality rate: 118/1000 live births

Health programmes

Immunization

Immunization coverage as well as the quality of services in Mongar district was considered far from satisfactory. Due to poor accessibility, services could not be extended throughout the district. Maternal and child health (MCH) clinics were limited to BHUs, as outreach clinics had not been established then. Services were irregular and poorly organized.

Lack of an efficient distribution system for vaccines and poor logistics led to frequent shortages and disruption of services. Only two BHUs were equipped with refrigerators. This meant that all the other BHUs had to obtain vaccines and logistic supplies from hospitals, irrespective of the distance from the hospital.

The immunization coverage for Mongar in 1985 was as follows: BCG 16%, measles 50%, DPT3 and OPV 52%.

Maternal health

Although no data are available, maternal morbidity and mortality in the district were probably high. This could be attributed to:

- A high prevalence of anaemia and malnutrition among this population group.
- Limited MCH services: out of 11 blocks, MCH services were available only in Mongar block.
- Low rates of skilled attendance at birth, low rates of hospital delivery: low antenatal and postnatal attendance in MCH clinics. Women preferred to deliver at home.
- Lack of female health workers: the role of male village health workers (VHWs) was limited when it came to attending deliveries, giving pre- and postnatal care and advising women.

Women in Mongar were never directly involved in development activities. Although they attended public meetings, their role was more or less limited to that of passive observers. Leading or initiating any community health development activities was a male-dominated area.

Communication and logistics support system

One of the major constraints in the district health-care delivery system was poor communication and poor management of drugs and logistics. Although the national highway traversed through the district and connected Mongar to the capital city and neighbouring districts, it touched very few villages making communication within the district very difficult. A walking distance of seven hours from one village to another is not unusual.

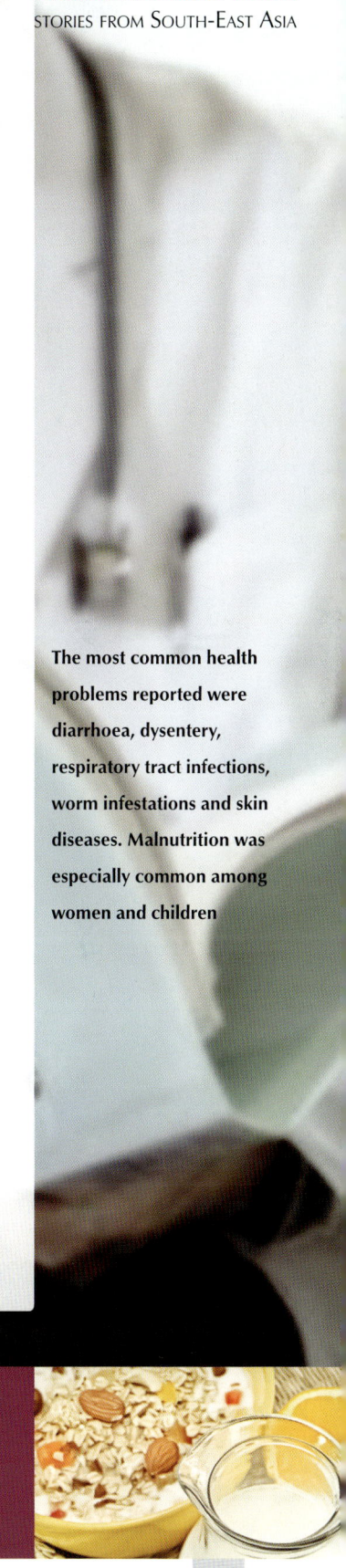

The most common health problems reported were diarrhoea, dysentery, respiratory tract infections, worm infestations and skin diseases. Malnutrition was especially common among women and children

> Women in Mongar were never directly involved in development activities. Although they attended public meetings, their role was more or less limited to that of passive observers. Leading or initiating any community health development activities was a male-dominated area

Mongar Health Services Development Project:
Bhutan: 1997 (Bhutan)

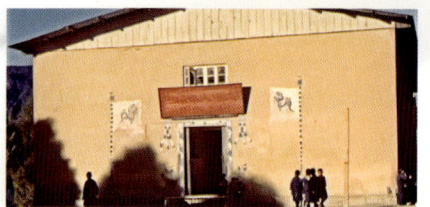
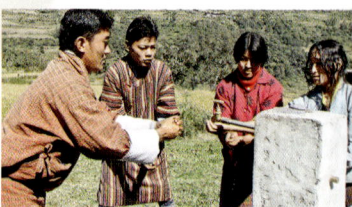

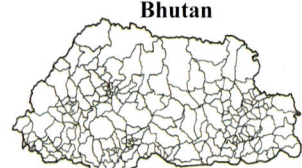

Bhutan

Poor communication and inefficient management and coordination hindered activities in the health units. Services were frequently disrupted due to lack of supplies of drugs and vaccines. An efficient and cost-effective mechanism for managing communication and logistic support to facilitate the smooth and efficient delivery of health services was found to be lacking.

Referral support system

Major obstacles were encountered with patient referrals due to poor communication. Social problems such as superstition and propaganda of traditional healers further obstructed timely referral. There was no system of feedback from the hospitals to peripheral health centres.

An efficient and cost-effective mechanism for managing communication and logistic support to facilitate the smooth and efficient delivery of health services was found to be lacking

5. The Mongar Health Services Development Project

The Mongar Health Services Development Project was launched with WHO support in 1985 and extended over a period of five years. As mentioned earlier, this project was implemented to maximize "Health for All by the year 2000" and community participation.

The main objectives were:

- To extend primary healthcare coverage to all people in the district, promote optimum utilization of services and raise the health status of the population;
- To establish a healthcare delivery system based on total community involvement at minimum cost, i.e. through utilization of available resources and appropriate technologies;
- To identify major health problems and develop appropriate interventions to reduce morbidity and mortality rates;
- To develop an effective support system (referral, logistics, communication and information);
- To promote intersectoral coordination as an integral component of community health development;
- To promote the adoption of the project in other districts.

5.1 Strategies adopted

- *Advocacy:* targeting district administrators, sectoral heads, district health workers and community leaders to garner their commitment to support implementation of the project activities at various levels of the district. The concept of one unified health delivery system encompassing promotive, preventive and curative measures was advocated.

- *Enhance intersectoral coordination:* through establishment of formal coordinating bodies at various levels of the operation with well-defined roles and responsibilities. Conforming with the principle of self reliance, utilize available resources, existing structures and technologies.

- *Community mobilization:* communities were involved at the planning stages to harness support for developing comprehensive health care in the district.

- *Expand coverage:* to improve accessibility and health infrastructure, sub-posts were constructed to support outreach activities, health centres relocated closer to local communities and existing health facilities consolidated.

- *Strengthen human resources for health:* volunteer village health workers (VVHWs) and female health volunteers were selected and recruited from local communities and their capacities built through regular training programmes.

- *Enhance knowledge, awareness and skills of rural communities:* provide health education on relevant health topics such as child care, nutrition, health and hygiene, disease and health hazards. Develop appropriate skills to bridge gaps between knowledge and practice.

- *Strengthen supervision and monitoring* at all levels.

- *Strengthen the communication and logistics support system to facilitate adequate supply:* reorganize the supply channel for

The Mongar Health Services Development Project was launched with WHO support in 1985 and extended over a period of five years

Communities were involved at the planning stages to harness support for developing comprehensive health care in the district

Mongar health services development project:
Bhutan: 1997 (Bhutan)

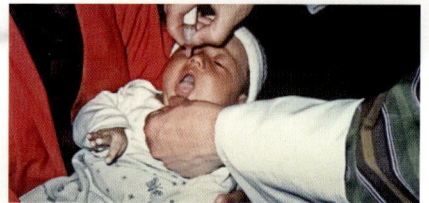
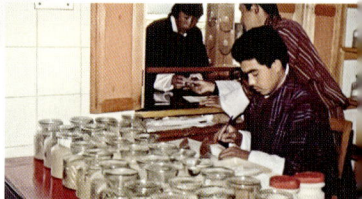

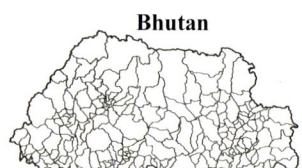
Bhutan

drugs, vaccines and logistics in the district, carry out a needs assessment of equipment and non-drug supplies in all district health centres, establish an efficient distribution and a buffer stock system in the district to replenish supplies, and ensure a mechanism to redistribute short-expiry drugs to centres requiring supplies.

5.2 Activities undertaken during the project period

- Advocacy, sensitization and education at various levels.
- Formation of organizing bodies and committees at various levels.
- Activities to improve sanitation.
  – Construction of pit latrines for safe disposal of excreta.
  – Shifting of pigsties and cattle sheds away from the house.
  – Building of refuse pits and improving overall cleanliness of the village.
- Activities to enhance community participation
  – Sensitization, orientation and education.
  – Selection and training of VVHWs.
  – Selection and training of women health workers in the area of MCH care.
- Relocation of health centres, construction and repair of existing health facilities.

5.3 Achievements and findings

Policy commitment

A major achievement of the project was the interlinking of all levels of decision-makers in the district. A District Health Committee was established to obtain policy commitment and functional cooperation in implementing the project. This committee was entrusted with the responsibility of deciding the feasibility of activities and coordinating assistance from other sectors. A technical committee was formed to advise on matters related to the development of

> A District Health Committee was established to obtain policy commitment and functional cooperation in implementing the project. This committee was entrusted with the responsibility of deciding the feasibility of activities and coordinating assistance from other sectors

project activities and facilitate urgent execution of activities. Local executive bodies were created to identify local problems, analyse the causes and make decisions to implement the required activities. This local body was crucial for promoting active participation and developing a self-sustaining community programme. The success of this local body stimulated the formation of a village development committee in all other districts in 1988.

Continuous support was forthcoming from local leaders. This support was instrumental in motivating communities to attend immunization sessions in MCH clinics, and increasing participation in community programmes such as sanitation and water supply, safe disposal of waste, health and hygiene.

Primary healthcare coverage

Primary healthcare services were expanded to all blocks of the district. Almost the entire population in Mongar District was covered within the five-year project period. About 100 farmers were elected by their communities and trained as VVHWs. They were initially trained for two weeks followed by refresher courses every six months. Their commitment and dedication was evident from the fact that there were no drop-outs, unlike the case in other districts. About 210 women were given one week's training in antenatal and postnatal care. This high coverage was attributed to the concerted efforts of health workers, VHWs and local leaders.

The concept of outreach clinics was first tried out in Mongar. Outreach clinics were established to increase coverage, facilitate health education and maximize opportunities for early detection of disease, its treatment and timely referral. The outreach clinics helped to bring health care as close as possible to the rural communities. By the end of the project period, 35 permanent outreach clinics were being run regularly from various BHUs and Mongar hospital.

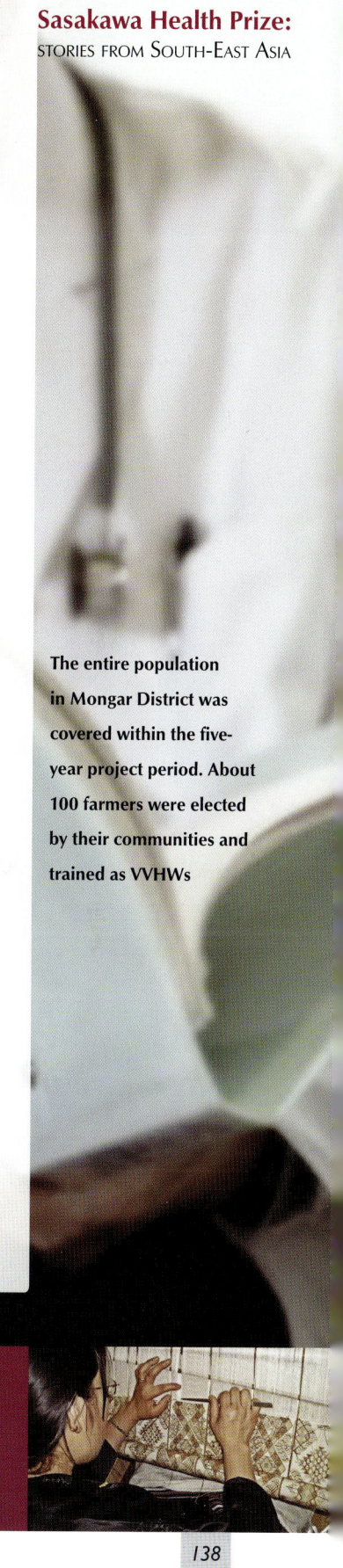

Sasakawa Health Prize:
STORIES FROM SOUTH-EAST ASIA

The entire population in Mongar District was covered within the five-year project period. About 100 farmers were elected by their communities and trained as VVHWs

Outreach clinics were established to increase coverage, facilitate health education and maximize opportunities for early detection of disease, its treatment and timely referral

MONGAR HEALTH SERVICES DEVELOPMENT PROJECT: BHUTAN: 1997 (BHUTAN)

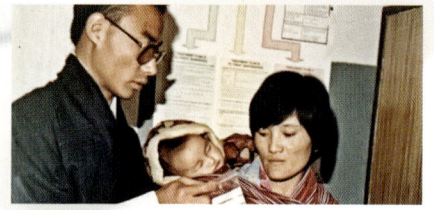
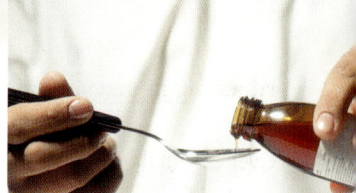
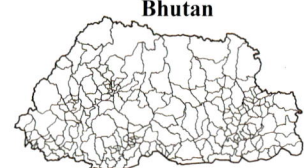

Bhutan

Health education was made an essential component of every MCH clinic. Rural communities were actively involved in constructing permanent outreach clinic sheds, and organizing and promoting the benefits of EPI services

Coverage of the Expanded Programme on Immunization (EPI) and growth monitoring

During the project implementation period, almost all BHUs were equipped with refrigerators and an efficient vaccine supply system was established. This greatly reduced the costs of transportation of vaccines. Health education was made an essential component of every MCH clinic. Rural communities were actively involved in constructing permanent outreach clinic sheds, and organizing and promoting the benefits of EPI services. About 300 women health workers were trained in the district to promote EPI in their communities.

Towards the end of the project, 94% of all children in Mongar district were fully immunized before the age of one year; 85% of the interviewed mothers could show their road-to-health card. Children were weighed six times on average after birth.

Nutrition

Almost all houses had kitchen gardens even before the start of the project. New varieties of vegetables and fruits were introduced during the project period. However, the lack of provision of seeds for the kitchen gardens was a major impediment to diversification of nutritional intake after the project period had ended.

Maternal health

About 70% of women received antenatal care and more than 75% of women had visited the antenatal clinic at least three to four times before delivery. About 85% of women were given two doses of tetanus toxoid (TT) and 95% received iron and folic acid. Almost half the women surveyed knew the benefits of antenatal care. However, despite the fact that 300 female health workers were trained in the district, 95% of mothers still delivered at home; 80% of these deliveries were conducted by relatives and only 20% were assisted by a trained female worker.

Sasakawa Health Prize: STORIES FROM SOUTH-EAST ASIA

Water supply and sanitation

Over 75% of the houses in Mongar district had access to a safe piped water supply as compared to 26% of the rural population in Bhutan. In almost half of the houses visited, the water supply, storage and management of waste products was found to be acceptable or good. About 94% of the houses had a latrine that was used by adults and children. About two thirds of the latrines were constructed after the start of the Mongar district health project.

The VVHWs were actively involved in protecting and maintaining rural water supply schemes. The respective Gewog development community was made responsible for assessing the rural water supply needs in the village.

Although cooperation and coordination for the rural water supply schemes were sought through the Gewog development committee, the health sector was of the view that they should be given the responsibility for planning and implementing the schemes in rural areas, as water supply and sanitation were essential elements of health care. Rural water supply schemes were handed over to the Health Department in 1998.

Knowledge, attitude and skills

The evaluation report revealed that:

- 85% of mothers recognized the oral rehydration solution (ORS) packets and 80% had used them. Of these, 87% knew how to prepare ORS. (A nationwide review on control of diarrhoeal diseases [CDD] revealed that the ORS access rate was 45% nationwide, 65% of mothers recognized an ORS packet, 59% had used it and 19% had prepared it correctly.)
- 50% of mothers could mention on an average at least three diseases prevented by immunization.
- 75% of the mothers were aware that weighing helped to monitor the growth of children or that it could help to see whether they had some disease.

The respective Gewog development community was made responsible for assessing the rural water supply needs in the village

Despite the fact that 300 female health workers were trained in the district, 95% of mothers still delivered at home; 80% of these deliveries were conducted by relatives and only 20% were assisted by a trained female worker

Mongar health services development project:
Bhutan: 1997 (Bhutan)

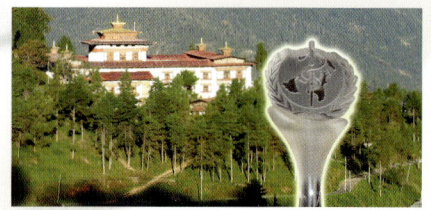
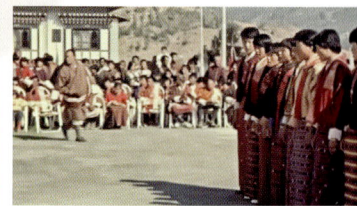

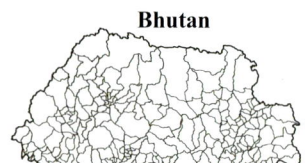

Cultural factors impeding the accessibility to health services were reduced drastically due to increased knowledge and awareness

Illness episodes and health-seeking behaviour

The disease frequency reported among 42 children during a period of two months showed that 65% of children had respiratory tract infections, 35% diarrhoea and others had skin infection, worm infestation, and diseases of the teeth and gums.

Only one quarter of these 42 children who were ill during the survey period were referred to the health facility, either by the VHW or by the health worker. Eight children were treated exclusively with home-made herbs. Seventy-five per cent of the mothers interviewed said that they first took their child to the health worker and the remaining said that they first visited a religious person.

Availability and accessibility of referral health services

Considering the rough terrain and the scattered location of the households, the project succeeded in bringing health care within an acceptable walking distance of the villages through relocation and construction of sub-posts in strategic areas. Services such as EPI and MCH were delivered on a monthly basis in geographically well-distributed subunits. Cultural factors impeding the accessibility to health services were reduced drastically due to increased knowledge and awareness.

Communities organized the transport of patients on stretchers to road points. From these points, transfer of patients was coordinated with the hospital ambulance service. Over the project period, the number of referrals from the communities to the hospital tripled and that to outpatient departments quadrupled.

A referral form was introduced to refer patients from the villages to the district hospitals. This allowed feedback to basic health workers and facilitated documentation of referrals. The district hospital was well equipped with drugs, laboratory services, an X-ray unit, and surgical, physical rehabilitation and community health services.

5.4 Lessons learned

1. District health development entails more than building health infrastructures, appointing health workers and opening mobile outreach clinics. In order to develop a health system and sustain it after external support is withdrawn, the active participation and commitment of the community is required. Activities initiated through community participation not only meet the local needs but also promote mobilization of community resources and ensure long-term viability.

2. VVHWs are an essential link between the community and the health system. They are a valuable resource for enhancing awareness and understanding of health and health problems. This system also integrates traditional values and beliefs into health-related activities.

3. Selection of the right person is the single most important element in the VVHW system. Village communities must understand the criteria for selection of a VHW and the expected roles and responsibilities. A person who is responsible and well respected by the community has more chances of being accepted and becoming a catalyst for change in that community. Candidates may be farmers, retired soldiers or lay monks.

4. An information system is an integral part of the health-care delivery system. Collection, analysis and dissemination of health information at all levels is vital. Information must be utilized at various levels to further improve services.

5. Rural development projects must involve all administrative levels of the district. Stakeholders must be involved during the planning stages if a project or programme is to succeed.

Activities initiated through community participation not only meet the local needs but also promote mobilization of community resources and ensure long-term viability

Communities organized the transport of patients on stretchers to road points. From these points, transfer of patients was coordinated with the hospital ambulance service

MONGAR HEALTH SERVICES
DEVELOPMENT PROJECT:
BHUTAN: 1997 (BHUTAN)

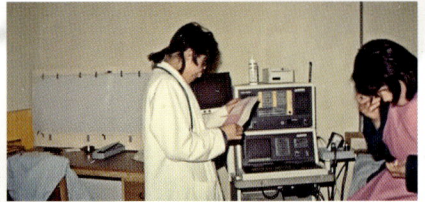 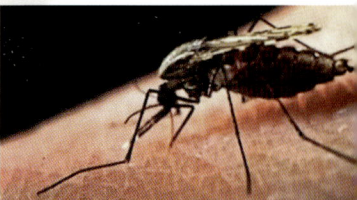

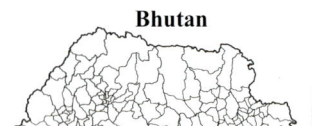
Bhutan

The Royal Government's effort was recognized internationally through the Sasakawa award to the Mongar Health Service in 1997

6. Pooling and use of common resources such as human resources for supervision, structures and transport greatly reduce the cost of services.

7. Support from local leaders and local bodies such as the village development committee is crucial for promoting active participation and developing a self-sustaining community programme.

6. Conclusion

Since 1961, the development of health services in Bhutan has been remarkable. The country progressed from a situation of practically no health infrastructure to a comprehensive network of services within a span of two decades. With the adoption of the primary health care system in 1979, an integrated, equitable and balanced health service consisting of a package of preventive, promotive, curative and rehabilitative services was established. The health status of the people has greatly improved through effective implementation of the eight essential elements of primary health care.

The Royal Government's effort was recognized internationally through the Sasakawa award to the Mongar Health Service in 1997. The success of the Mongar Health Services Development Project is largely attributable to the support and commitment at the district policy level, active participation of the local communities and unstinting support of international partners, in particular, WHO. The lessons learned from the Mongar District Health Project were applied to other districts to improve the national healthcare delivery system.

7. Epilogue

Today, over 90% of the Bhutanese population has access to primary healthcare services. About two thirds of this population now lives within three hours' walking distance from the nearest health facility.

The healthcare service in Bhutan is delivered through a four-tiered network consisting of a national and two regional referral hospitals, 29 district hospitals, 181 basic health units (BHUs) and 518 outreach clinics. More than 1200 VHWs have been trained in the country and actively contribute to increasing health coverage of rural populations. The need to ensure active community participation prompted the health sector to decentralize many of its programmes to the district hospitals. With the exception of referral hospitals, training institutes and medical supplies, all hospitals are placed under the district administration.

Along with expansion of infrastructure, human resource development has also taken a big turn over time. As a result, the quality and efficiency of delivery of healthcare services have been enhanced. The information available puts the ratio of doctors for every 10 000 population at 1.7, which is a significant improvement in the context of Bhutan's development. Even so, there is a need to further develop human resources, especially at the more specialized levels.

The emphasis now lies on reaching the unreached population and further improving the quality of services at all levels. Bhutan is well on track to achieve the Millennium Development Goals (MDGs). This is largely attributable to the farsighted development strategies of the past 40 years.

The healthcare service in Bhutan is delivered through a four-tiered network consisting of a national and two regional referral hospitals, 29 district hospitals, 181 basic health units (BHUs) and 518 outreach clinics

Since 1961, the development of health services in Bhutan has been remarkable. The country progressed from a situation of practically no health infrastructure to a comprehensive network of services within a span of two decades

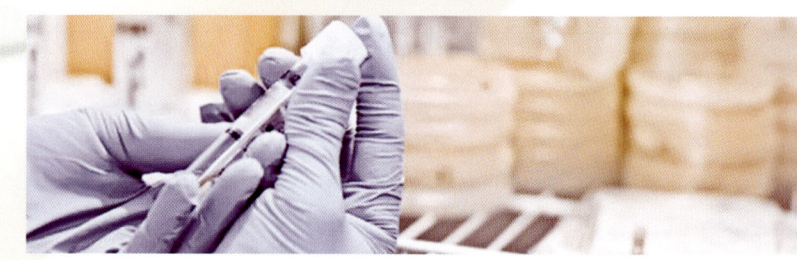

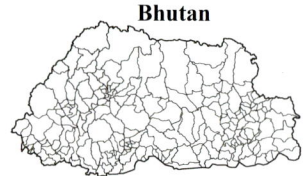
Bhutan

8. Bibliography

1. *The Fifth Plan Program for Mongar District (1981–86/87). Thimphu: Department of Information, 1981.*

2. *Royal Government of Bhutan, Central Statistical Office, Planning Commission. Statistical handbook of Bhutan 1986. Thimphu. 1987.*

3. *de Jong JTVM.* **Assignment report** *on e***valuation of Mongar project, Bhutan, 1-21 November 1988. New Delhi: WHO Regional Office for South-East Asia,** *1989. http://repository.searo.who.int/handle/123456789/11893 - accessed 17 May 2012.*

4. *Tenzin, Sonam, Dorji Rinchen. Mongar Health Services Development Project. Thimphu: Health Division, Ministry of Health & Education, 1996.*

5. *Declaration of Alma-Ata International Conference on Primary Health Care. Alma-Ata, USSR, 6–12 September 1978. http://www.who.int/hpr/NPH/docs/declaration_almaata.pdf - accessed 11 November 2011.*

6. *Royal Government of Bhutan. First Five-Year Plan 1961–66. Thimphu, 1961. http://www.gnhc.gov.bt/wp-content/uploads/2011/04/1stFYP.pdf - accessed 14 May 2012.*

7. *Royal Government of Bhutan. Second Five-Year Plan 1966–1971. Thimphu, 1966. http://www.gnhc.gov.bt/wp-content/uploads/2011/04/02fyp.pdf - accessed 14 May 2012.*

8. *Royal Government of Bhutan. Third Five-Year Plan 1971–1976. Thimphu, 1971. http://www.gnhc.gov.bt/wp-content/uploads/2011/04/03fyp.pdf - accessed 14 May 2012.*

9. Royal Government of Bhutan, Planning Commission. Fourth Five-Year Plan: half yearly progress report for the period from 1.4.77 to 30.9.77. Thimphu, 1977.

10. Royal Government of Bhutan. Fifth Five-Year Plan, 1981–87. Thimphu, 1982. http://www.gnhc.gov.bt/wp-content/uploads/2011/04/05fyp.pdf - accessed 14 May 2012.

11. Royal Government of Bhutan, Ministry of Health. Health sector review, Bhutan. Thimphu, Ministry of Health, February 2007.

12. New Zealand, Ministry of Health. Public Health in a Primary Health Care Setting. Wellington, 2003.

13. Stapleton M. Bhutan Essential Drugs Programme: a case history. New Delhi, WHO Department of Essential Drugs and Medicines Policy, 2000.

14. Druk Medical Journal. 1986 volume 2.

15. Royal Government of Bhutan. Millennium Development Goals. Progress Report 2005. Thimphu: 2005.

16. Royal Government of Bhutan, Gross National Happiness Commission. Tenth Five-Year Plan. 2008-2013 (Volume 1 and Volume 2). Thimphu, 2009. http://www.gnhc.gov.bt/wp-content/uploads/2011/10thplan/TenthPlan_Vol1_Web.pdf and http://www.gnhc.gov.bt/wp-content/uploads/2011/10thplan/TenthPlan_Vol2_Web.pdf - accessed 14 May 2012.

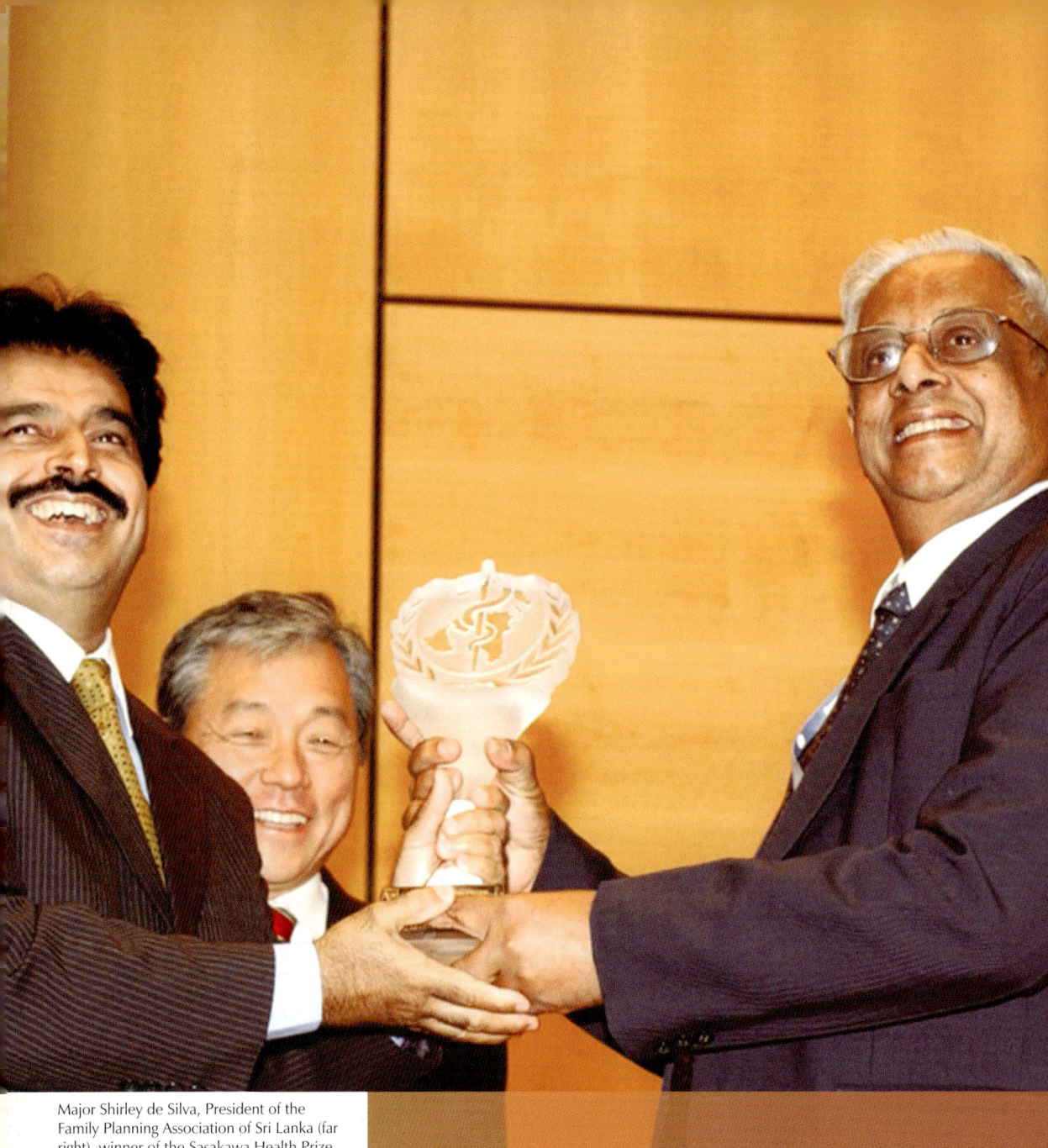

Major Shirley de Silva, President of the Family Planning Association of Sri Lanka (far right), winner of the Sasakawa Health Prize receiving the 2004 Sasakawa Health Prize from Mr M.N Khan of Pakistan, president of the 57th World Health Assembly.

Photo credit:
WHO/Pierre Virot

CHAPTER 10

2004

The triumphant journey of FPA Sri Lanka: Sasakawa and beyond [*]

Recipient:
The Family Planning Association of Sri Lanka
(Sri Lanka)

[*] Draft prepared by Mrs Sabina Omar
Family Planning Association of Sri Lanka, Bullers Lane, Colombo 7, Sri Lanka

T he Family Planning Association of Sri Lanka (FPA) is a pioneering organization that has defined the landscape of family planning and sexual and reproductive health (SRH) in Sri Lanka

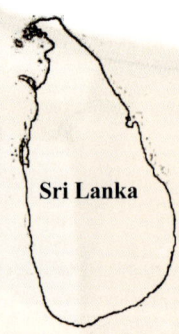

Sri Lanka

During the post-Independence era, family planning issues did not feature on the government's "to do" list. The population had doubled between 1900 and 1948

1. Introduction

The Family Planning Association of Sri Lanka (FPA) is a pioneering organization that has defined the landscape of family planning and sexual and reproductive health (SRH) in Sri Lanka. From its inception, the organization has experienced a journey of challenges and achievements; above all, the organization has witnessed a shift in perceptions.

After four centuries of colonial rule, Sri Lanka gained independence in 1948. Many sexual health and social issues needed to be addressed. Poverty, nutrition, and access to health services were intrinsically linked issues affecting the well-being of the population. During this post-Independence era, family planning issues did not feature on the government's "to do" list. The population had doubled between 1900 and 1948. The numbers of infant and maternal deaths were high. An increase in the population at a macro level and families affected by infant/maternal mortality at the micro level existed side by side.

Prior to the 1950s, family planning and reproductive health were seldom discussed by the government or in the public sphere. The multireligious social make-up of the country also contributed to diverse views on family planning and sexuality. Further, family planning did not feature in the government health plans of the time. The FPA has been at the forefront of family planning services, support and education, introducing new and innovative concepts relating to SRH in Sri Lanka. Reaching out to people in need of support and gaining their trust has been essential in the journey of the FPA in order to bring family planning to the fore as a lifestyle choice. The concept had to be liberated from the many taboos associated with family planning and sexual relationships.

2. The concept of family planning and pioneering steps

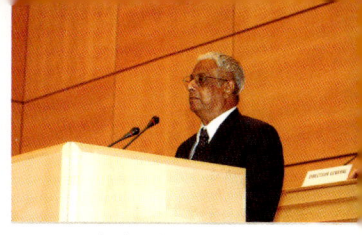

Major Shirley de Silva, President of the Family Planning Association of Sri Lanka addressing the 57th World Health Assembly.

Photo credit: WHO/Pierre Virot

The journey of the FPA began with the small steps taken by a group of friends and acquaintances consisting of professionals and social workers, who discussed the feasibility of starting a family planning association in Ceylon – as Sri Lanka was then known. Following informal discussions, an inaugural meeting of the FPA was held on 15 January 1953. At the outset, volunteers were responsible for all the activities of the association. Staff support was enlisted only in the fifth year. The primary objective of the association at the time was to establish family planning service delivery centres or clinics in different parts of the country. The lack of funds limited the number of clinics.

New life was injected into the Association in 1954 when it became an affiliate of the International Planned Parenthood Federation (IPPF). The association also received funds from the Swedish government to acquire the necessary equipment and contraceptive support to expand its service base. These pioneering steps impacted the demographic course of Sri Lanka. Even before the sexual revolution of the 1960s, the need for SRH services, especially for young women of reproductive age, was a cause espoused by the organization. In 1970, the organization was formally incorporated as the Family Planning Association of Ceylon. With the introduction of the country's first Republican Constitution in 1972, the country was christened Sri Lanka, and the organization changed its name to the Family Planning Association of Sri Lanka in 1974. Today, although still incorporated under this name, the organization has gained prominence and acceptance as FPA Sri Lanka (FPA).

Reaching out to people in need of support and gaining their trust has been essential in the journey of the FPA in order to bring family planning to the fore as a lifestyle choice

In the early days of the FPA, the task at hand was not merely handing out popular contraceptives. Starting at the grass-roots level, the need of the moment was to create awareness and educate young men and women about individual choices and provide the best for their children and families. The ability to make choices relating to sexuality, one's body and the size of one's family translated to improved nutrition, care, education, and a better quality of life for parents and

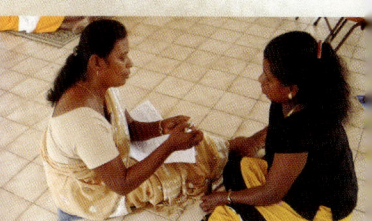

With the introduction of the country's first Republican Constitution in 1972, the country was christened Sri Lanka, and the organization changed its name to the Family Planning Association of Sri Lanka in 1974

The triumphant journey of FPA Sri Lanka: Sasakawa and beyond: 2004 (Sri Lanka)

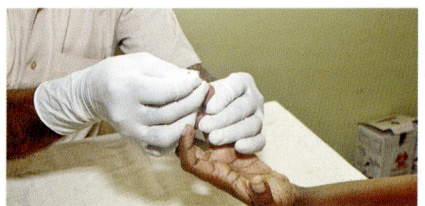
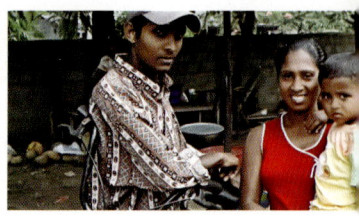

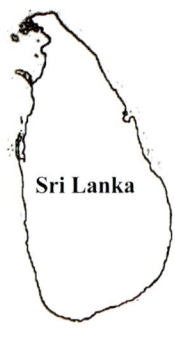

Over the past 57 years, the country has experienced a demographic shift. The growth rates during the first half of the twentieth century saw the population heading towards dangerously unsustainable numbers

children alike. The mental anguish of a family caused by infant and maternal mortality could be reduced. More importantly, the physical and psychological trauma experienced by women who have multiple births could be minimized. The services provided by the FPA gave people the tools to improve their quality of life. The FPA's message was focused on an improved sense of well-being for families. Through its ground-breaking first steps, the FPA laid the foundation for policy decisions by the Government of Sri Lanka (GOSL) relating to fertility, thereby reducing the high rates of maternal and infant mortality, and improving the health and nutrition of mothers and children. Today, these efforts have paid rich dividends.

3. A demographic shift through family planning

Over the past 57 years, the country has experienced a demographic shift. The growth rates during the first half of the twentieth century saw the population heading towards dangerously unsustainable numbers. However, due to the efforts of the FPA and support by the GOSL, the country sees stabilization in population growth. Although population stabilization was not on the agenda of the FPA, the work done with the community in relation to family planning and sexual health has indirectly contributed to this demographic shift. Within one year, the GOSL recognized the untiring initial steps of the FPA to improve the quality of life through family planning. The advantages of moving towards a sustainable and stable population as a developing nation were also recognized. Provision was made for an annual grant of Rs 2500 to the FPA in the 1954/55 government budget.

During the early years, the FPA established family planning clinics around the country served by trained doctors, nurses and midwives. They also visited government medical institutions to initiate clinical services. The FPA won the support of medical staff, who voluntarily provided their services. Going beyond providing clinical services, the FPA worked to gain the trust of the people through discussions, education and interaction with the public. The initiatives of the FPA prompted the GOSL to integrate family planning into the Health Ministry's Maternal and Child Health Programme in 1965. Subsequently, the

GOSL stepped in and acquired the majority of clinics operated by the FPA. This was a definitive step, whereby fertility and family planning entered the mainstream health services of the country.

Family planning is a culturally sensitive subject in a multi-ethnic and multireligious society. The FPA had to create space for dialogue on a platform of mutual understanding. The FPA first reached out to those in dire need of SRH services and support. Easing itself into the psyche of the people, the FPA gathered momentum as a positive force, gradually gaining wider acceptance by the average Sri Lankan.

The International Conference on Population and Development (held in Cairo in 1994) changed the paradigm of family planning with the focus shifting to SRH the world over. Access to SRH was recognized as a right, and ensuring universal access to SRH by 2015 was a part of the Millennium Development Goals. The GOSL adopted a National Population Policy in 1989/90, which was redefined by way of a second policy in 1998 – the Population and Reproductive Health Policy. Though started as a family planning organization, the FPA adapted to the global trends and Sri Lankan goals in reproductive health care.

4. Breaking new ground in the area of contraceptives

In the 1950s, the only methods of contraception available were the barrier methods (condom and diaphragm); spermicides were introduced soon after. In 1963, the intrauterine device (IUD) was introduced by the FPA and, in 1968, the three-monthly injection Depo Provera. The FPA also provided sterilization in the form of vasectomies and tubectomies, if desired by the client. The introduction of each method of contraception and creating awareness about the right to choose and access contraception were all ground-breaking initiatives. However, the introduction of the oral contraceptive pill (the pill) in 1960 followed by clinical trials transformed the lives of women and men in an unprecedented manner. The pill proved to be the most popular contraceptive in the 1960s, together with the IUD.

> **The FPA also provided sterilization in the form of vasectomies and tubectomies, if desired by the client. The introduction of each method of contraception and creating awareness about the right to choose and access contraception were all ground-breaking initiatives**

> Family planning is a culturally sensitive subject in a multi-ethnic and multi-religious society. The FPA had to create space for dialogue on a platform of mutual understanding

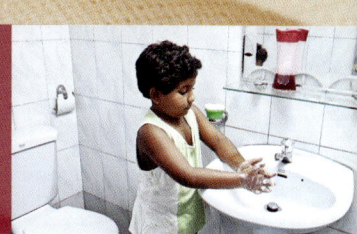

THE TRIUMPHANT JOURNEY
OF FPA SRI LANKA:
SASAKAWA AND BEYOND:
2004 (SRI LANKA)

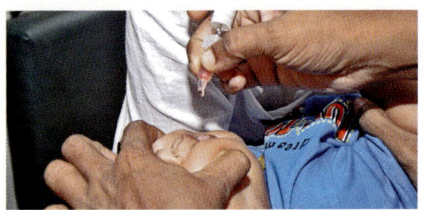
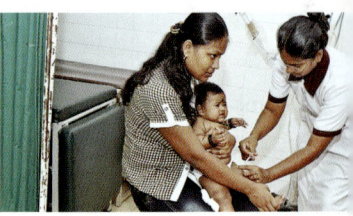

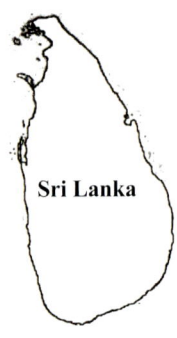

Sri Lanka

Contraceptives have empowered women in Sri Lanka from all ethnic and religious backgrounds to plan their own lives and that of their children

The FPA worked to move contraceptives from under the shroud of suspicion and taboo through provision of much-needed information, education and communication. Contraceptives have empowered women in Sri Lanka from all ethnic and religious backgrounds to plan their own lives and that of their children. This has provided more women in Sri Lanka the opportunity for stable employment, education and the ability to focus on the health, nutrition, education and well-being of their children and families. The availability of contraceptives has also resulted in women delaying childbirth. The increase in the number of women giving birth above the age of 30 years is evidence of this. While the pill has impacted women on a personal level, it has also shaped the way the country has moved forward, with more women empowered to contribute to the economy and the next generation, whether as a part of the workforce or as caregivers equipped to provide the best support to their families.

The FPA took the unprecedented step of introducing the emergency contraceptive pill – Postinor 2 – to the Sri Lankan public. The project was funded by The Consortium for Emergency Contraception and was launched in 1997. The goal was to introduce a branded, dedicated emergency contraceptive pill (ECP) to the local market. The FPA conducted aggressive educational campaigns and created awareness among health workers and the public. All SRH training seminars as well as the mainstream media provided information about the ECP. The manner in which the ECP works was communicated and the FPA took steps to ensure that the message was clear: the ECP, if administered properly, would not amount to an abortion, the side-effects were minimal and it was not a method of contraception. At the outset, Postinor 2 was available only through private medical practitioners. The FPA facilitated the opening of several thousands of Postinor 2 sales outlets throughout the country. The product was made available through the pharmaceutical network in the country as part of the project. The creation of awareness and increased accessibility delivered results, as sales reached an average of 18 000 packets per month by the end of 2002. By 2003, over 3000 pharmacies were purchasing the product from FPA marketing officers and it was clear that the product had gained popularity as a brand and as a reliable emergency contraceptive.

As the use of the ECP was a relatively new concept for the public, the FPA created a safe and reliable space for discussion through a "hotline" in October 1997, which proved to be one of the most effective tools of communication. The hotline was promoted through advertising campaigns for Postinor 2 and was operative from 8 am to 5 pm on all working days of the week. It was an unparalleled success. At the time, on average, the hotline received 30 calls per day from people in all parts of Sri Lanka. From the nature of the calls and callers, the FPA gleaned information on the target groups and how to better serve them. It was also evident that the advice sought was not limited to the ECP but also included topics such as sexual health and family planning. The anonymity of the hotline ensured privacy.

5. Sensitizing the media

The media is a powerful tool for creating awareness on health and reproductive issues among the public. The FPA conducted a two-day residential workshop for media personnel in 1998. Members of the print and electronic media participated in the programme, which featured lectures and films on human sexuality, reproductive health, family planning, sexually transmitted infections (STIs) and AIDS. Following this programme, a large number of articles were published in popular newspapers and journals on SRH issues. In addition, the doctors of the FPA were featured on radio and TV programmes and gave interviews, which gave the FPA publicity, and a face and voice though which to reach out to the public.

The FPA conducted aggressive educational campaigns and created awareness among health workers and the public

The search for new methods to communicate led the FPA to produce a full-length film entitled Yuvathipathi (man and wife), which premiered in July 1994. The film saw full houses at each of the three showings during the first few weeks across all 13 cinemas in the country. The Regal Cinema in Colombo showed the film continuously for 92 days, breaking their highest collection record up till then. The film was shown with English subtitles in some cinemas to attract non-Sinhala speaking cinemagoers. This was the first commercial film with family planning and reproductive health information produced by a South

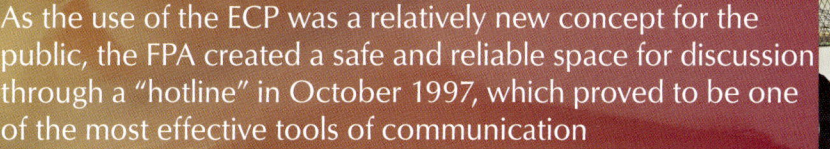

As the use of the ECP was a relatively new concept for the public, the FPA created a safe and reliable space for discussion through a "hotline" in October 1997, which proved to be one of the most effective tools of communication

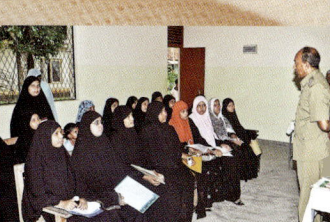

The triumphant journey of FPA Sri Lanka: Sasakawa and beyond: 2004 (Sri Lanka)

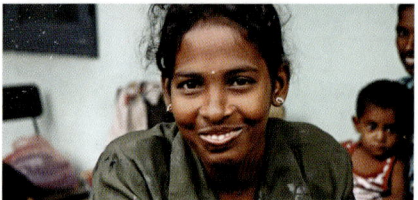 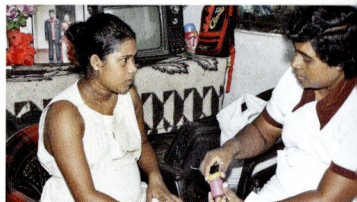

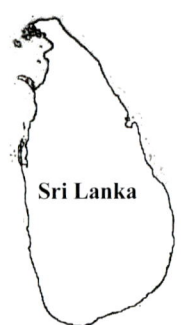

The FPA provided training for salespeople and distributors on SRH issues to ensure that the retailers would understand the needs of their customers

Asian country. Appreciated by both critics and the audience, the film grossed the second-highest collection for films shown in the year 1995. The National Film Corporation forwarded the film to film festivals in India and China. It was also nominated for prestigious film awards in Sri Lanka and reached a wider audience in a manner that was well received by the target groups.

6. Taking proactive steps

6.1 Ensuring the accessibility of contraceptives

Even after the introduction of contraceptive methods such as the pill. the challenge of accessibility remained. The innovative Contraceptive Retail Sales marketing programme of the FPA, introduced during the latter part of the 1970s, played a pivotal role in making contraceptives available from trustworthy and reliable sources at affordable prices. The FPA promoted the availability of a choice of condoms and contraceptive pills. A condom by the brand name "Preethi" (meaning joy or happiness) and an oral contraceptive pill named "Mithuri" (female friend) are two trusted brands used by many women and men in the country today due to market penetration, affordability and visibility. The FPA worked to create a successful sales network through retailers and pharmacies throughout the country. The FPA provided training for salespeople and distributors on SRH issues to ensure that the retailers would understand the needs of their customers. They would also communicate these details to the FPA, thereby assisting the FPA to improve the programme and the contraceptive sales services offered. For example, what should be done if a 12-year-old boy wished to purchase a condom? Could the retail salesperson refuse to sell? The FPA created awareness among the retailers of the consequences of not using a condom, which could result in tragedy for the boy and his young partner.

Advertising campaigns including billboards in prominent locations and panels placed in shop fronts were used to create visibility for brands such as Preethi and Mithuri. This programme supplemented the GOSL's efforts to distribute contraceptives through clinics and midwives during home visits. While this provided an essential service, it also resulted in revenue generation for the organization. Today, the contraceptive pill and condoms are freely available in supermarkets and pharmacies around the country and the pill is available to women without a prescription.

6.2 Increasing the use of contraceptives

The Praja Shanthi (Bliss to the community) Family Planning and Reproductive Health Education and Motivational Project was launched in 1990. The main aim of the project was to achieve replacement-level fertility by the year 2000. This project contributed toward a national goal in a sustainable manner while promoting reproductive health in underserved areas. The project was implemented around the country with the support of six other NGOS and mobilized grass-roots level volunteers to spearhead SRH educational activities including through home visits. Leaders were trained to take on leadership at the community level. Education was provided on family planning, health, gender issues, women's empowerment, and contraceptives, and awareness programmes for the youth. Praja Shanthi had a direct impact on the increase in the levels of SRH awareness among youth, an increase in the use of contraceptives by married couples, and also addressed the general health status of the people in the project areas. Working from within the community created a rapport between the FPA volunteers and the community. This project thrived on the spirit of volunteerism and the energy and dedication of the youth. It attracted the commitment of village leaders as they recognized the numerous benefits to the people of their community. Each year, the project worked in different areas of the country and trained new volunteers to spearhead Praja Shanthi activities within communities. The project resulted in improved contraceptive prevalence rates in the project areas and the FPA was able to meet its objectives by project completion in 1999. As recorded in the FPA annual report of 1998–1999, for the year under review, the project was implemented in 40 midwife areas in four districts of the country; 518 trained grass-roots level volunteers reached a population of over 120 000. The average contraceptive prevalence rates increased from 48% to 79%. These volunteers undertook 100 700 home visits. This highlights the reach of the project, and its penetration and acceptance within communities.

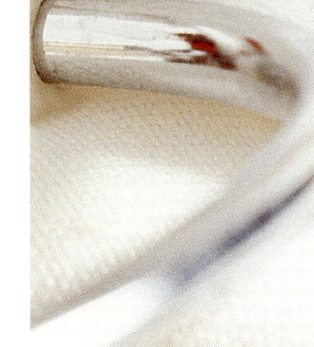

This project thrived on the spirit of volunteerism and the energy and dedication of the youth. It attracted the commitment of village leaders as they recognized the numerous benefits to the people of their community

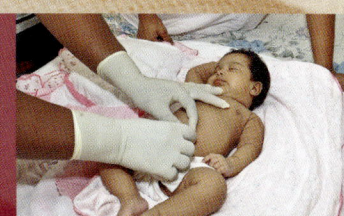

The Praja Shanthi (Bliss to the community) Family Planning and Reproductive Health Education and Motivational Project was launched in 1990. The main aim of the project was to achieve replacement-level fertility by the year 2000

The triumphant journey of FPA Sri Lanka: Sasakawa and beyond: 2004 (Sri Lanka)

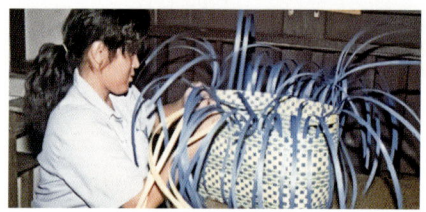
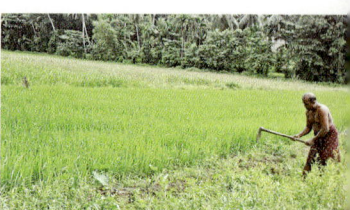

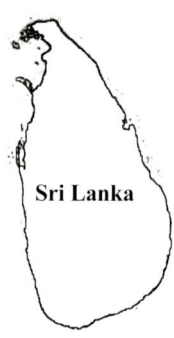

Sri Lanka

The FPA has conducted advocacy programmes in an effort to educate the public and abolish the traditional "virginity test", which has to be humiliatingly endured by a new bride

6.3 Women's health

The FPA recognized the need to start a Well Woman Clinic to encourage women to have routine health checks as, after childbirth, the average woman neglected her health. This service is conducted daily at the FPA headquarters in Colombo. The clinic is conducted by a team of lady doctors. Through this programme, which was initiated in 1997, women are given a complete physical and gynaecological examination in addition to blood and urine examinations and a Pap smear test. Clients are provided with the test results and reports and, where required, referred to consultants for special investigations. In 2002, 18 609 clients were seen at the clinic. This clinic also offers much-needed counselling services for clients with sexual problems such as impotence, non-consummation of marriage, frigidity, lack of sexual desire, etc. Another area where counselling is required is where newly-wed couples – especially women – have to prove their virginity at the time of marriage. The FPA has conducted advocacy programmes in an effort to educate the public and abolish the traditional "virginity test", which has to be humiliatingly endured by a new bride. The negative impact of such a traumatic experience on women, virginity and the sexual rights of women are included in all FPA reproductive health education programmes. Proactive action is necessary to create a change in traditional perceptions that degrade women and their sexual rights.

The FPA has from its inception worked with couples on subfertility issues. At the FPA's Subfertility Clinic, couples can discuss fertility issues, seek guidance while the FPA conducts investigations and suggests solutions and treatment for subfertility. In 2002, 625 couples registered for these services and 77 previously subfertile women conceived and delivered during the year.

Sasakawa Health Prize:
STORIES FROM SOUTH-EAST ASIA

6.4 Empowering women

The services provided by the FPA would be immaterial if women were not aware of their rights and their ability to make decisions that impact their daily lives. With a view to creating this awareness and empowering women through education and new perspectives, the FPA launched the Mahila Shanthi – Gender Equity and Empowerment Project – in 1997 to "empower women for a better tomorrow". The project was delivered through influential and respected members of the community at the village level and also directly to the target groups. The focus of the programme was to sensitize women to their rights and responsibilities, while aiming at attitudinal changes that are crucial in a sociocultural context. Women were made aware of the different roles played by them as mothers, wives, daughters, sisters and employees, and their rights in each of these roles. This initiative was necessary in a social context where women are traditionally expected to partake of their meal after the male members of the family. This places the already undernourished pregnant or lactating woman at a higher health risk. Similarly, depriving the girl child of nutrition would lead to future health and reproductive complications that affect the next generation: an endless vicious cycle that has many women in its grip. Stereotypical gender roles see women as passive, tolerant, non-aggressive home makers who are subject to violence and abuse within the home when they are not empowered to speak for themselves and assert their rights and make their voices heard. This project opened a window for many women, giving them the power of choice. Many males who participated in the Mahila Shanthi programmes agreed that women have equal rights and that the programme was a good "eye-opener" for them.

Aware of its responsibility to uphold gender equity, a male reproductive health service was introduced by the FPA in 1998. During this special weekly clinic, a consultant doctor was available to provide advice and treatment to men who suffered from SRH issues. Men have also been given the opportunity to speak up and voice their concerns, especially in relation to issues such as impotence, virility and libido, and sexual health issues such as testicular cancer, sterilization and AIDS.

> **Women were made aware of the different roles played by them as mothers, wives, daughters, sisters and employees, and their rights in each of these roles**

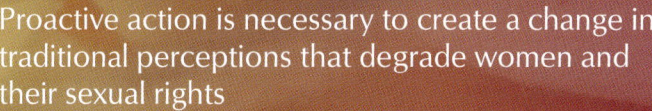

Proactive action is necessary to create a change in traditional perceptions that degrade women and their sexual rights

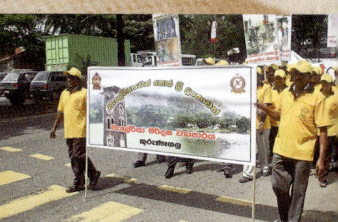

THE TRIUMPHANT JOURNEY
OF FPA SRI LANKA:
SASAKAWA AND BEYOND:
2004 (SRI LANKA)

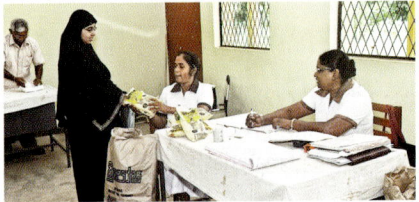
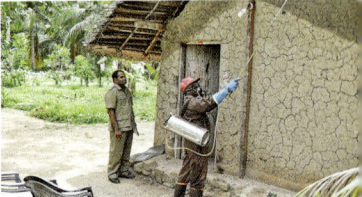

7. Reaching out to neglected populations

Throughout its journey, the FPA has reached out to social groups on the fringes of society and brought to light the issues faced by these diverse social groups. A few examples of the extensive work carried out by the FPA are given below.

7.1 The youth

At the beginning of the FPA's work, it was evident that discussion of sexual health and related issues was limited. Young people would be exposed to information that was inaccurate, derogatory of women and sexual relations, and they continued to be in the dark regarding contraception and prevention of communicable diseases.

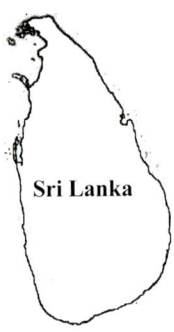

The organization took an innovative step in engaging the youth in counselling programmes as far back as 30 years ago – when counselling itself was an unknown concept for the average Sri Lankan

The FPA recognized the importance of counselling on sexual health and reproduction – this was necessary to create increased awareness and provide a safe space for dialogue on issues faced by adolescents and young adults. The organization took an innovative step in engaging the youth in counselling programmes as far back as 30 years ago – when counselling itself was an unknown concept for the average Sri Lankan. The counselling initiatives of the FPA took on greater significance because of the perception of youth during the early 1970s. The country had seen a youth insurgency in 1971 and there was much stigma and negative attitudes associated with any youth movement and activity. The FPA established what was known as the Tharuna Janagahana Kamituwa (Youth Division) in 1975 with the objective of creating awareness. These youth discussed SRH issues and carried out peer counselling.

Projects were crafted to disseminate information on various aspects of population, sexuality and reproduction among the youth of Sri Lanka, and to inculcate the idea that planned parenthood was important for a happy life. The FPA arranged for training and orientation for the members of the youth group in subjects such as population, family health and nutrition, communication, family planning, human reproduction, youth needs and aspirations, and planning and implementation of programmes. With the

159

Sasakawa Health Prize:
STORIES FROM SOUTH-EAST ASIA

support of the FPA, the Youth Division worked on educational seminars and programmes around the country. Active participation of the youth around the country was sought through campaigns such as a poster competition held in 1976. Over 75% of the entries had come from rural areas; thus, the awareness initiatives of the Youth Division and its Youth Committees had gained the trust of schools in rural areas. This was a great achievement as educating the youth of rural areas was one of the aims of the Youth Division. In 1976, a drama called "Prashna" (Problem) was staged to create awareness about the problems of overpopulation and raise funds for future youth-focused activities. Greeting cards were also designed by two members of the Youth Division to raise funds and popularize the two-child family norm.

The FPA also established a hotline to answer any questions on SRH issues. The overwhelming response to the hotline made it clear that more awareness and education on SRH issues was required. The FPA adopted a three-pronged approach in schools, focusing on education, counselling and provision of services. In 2001, with a view to improving knowledge on SRH issues among schoolchildren, a baseline survey was conducted in 40 schools to obtain information on the level of knowledge among adolescent schoolchildren on SRH issues.

Youth Clubs were another method used to create a platform for dialogue, support and the creation of awareness among students. Each Youth Club was set up in a classroom specially dedicated to the cause, and the club premises would carry posters with SRH information and audiovisual equipment that would facilitate learning. The principal of each school was appointed the patron of the club. Office bearers such as the president, secretary, etc. were appointed and provided with comprehensive training in leadership and decision-making skills. A question box placed within the club premises encouraged students to post questions and issues that could be addressed via discussions with peers and counsellors. Parents, teachers and the principals of participating schools have acknowledged the positive influence of the

> **Youth Clubs were another method used to create a platform for dialogue, support and the creation of awareness among students**

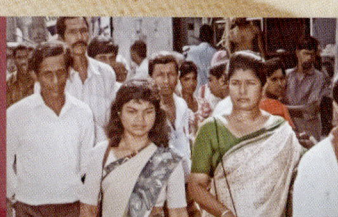

> Projects were crafted to disseminate information on various aspects of population, sexuality and reproduction among the youth of Sri Lanka, and to inculcate the idea that planned parenthood was important for a happy life

The Triumphant Journey of FPA Sri Lanka: Sasakawa and Beyond: 2004 (Sri Lanka)

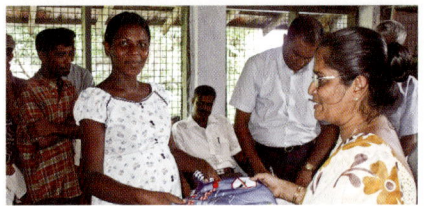 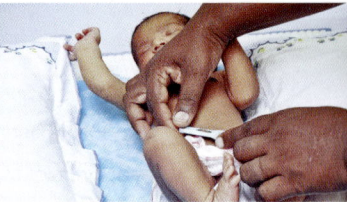

An annual interschool debate competition was another way in which young people were encouraged to engage in SRH issues

availability of information and counselling services. The creation of health awareness, and moving SRH beyond the realms of the taboo have resulted in teachers, who were previously reluctant to teach SRH in school for various reasons, gaining the confidence to teach the subject and discuss issues and questions posed by students in a comfortable environment. An annual inter-school debate competition was another way in which young people were encouraged to engage in SRH issues.

The Youth Caravan project focused on SRH awareness and education for adolescents by young people known as Youth Volunteer Members. This project was launched during the latter half of 1999 under the name "Youwana Yathra" (Youth Caravan). The main objective was the provision of knowledge on SRH issues to 15 000 youth with a view to encouraging them to be more responsible for their own SRH behaviour. Young people in the 16–25 years' age group volunteered their time and efforts, and received extensive training in leadership, counselling and communication skills. Based in Colombo and in other towns and cities around the country, the project worked towards maximum outreach. The project focused on five areas of SRH – STIs, AIDS and safe sex, unwanted pregnancies and abortion, sexual abuse and gender equality. The activities included seminars using audiovisual aids and interactive methods such as role-plays and discussions for youth who had completed their secondary education. Competitions and special activities such as dramas on days such as World AIDS Day, Population Day and even Valentine's Day were designed to create interest among the target groups.

The Reproductive Health Education Programme for Adolescents in Sri Lanka was first initiated by the FPA in 1982. This began with a programme called "Facts of Life" designed specifically for adolescents and implemented by Dr Sriani Basnayake, the Medicinal Director of the FPA. It proved to be extremely popular with parents who were looking for ways to provide guidance on the subject to their children. In 1984, the FPA began a wider programme on reproductive health in schools with the approval of the Minister of Education. Although reproductive health is a part of the school curriculum in the higher grades, the transfer of knowledge is not always successful as teachers do not have adequate knowledge or skills required to teach the subject. In 2002, a permanent Sexual and Reproductive Health Resource Centre to provide SRH knowledge to youth was set up at the FPA headquarters to bridge this gap and create a space for young people to learn without fear or embarrassment. A group of 10 young persons were trained as guides. This centre is open to schoolchildren and young people from all over the country. The centre helped to strengthen peer educational activities on SRH issues at the FPA and serves as a resource for school and educational authorities to educate teachers and students. It is also a training facility for other organizations engaged in youth educational activities. The FPA moved beyond posters and brochures and provided audiovisual information using modern technology in an effort to make the subject matter more tangible and less alien to young people.

7.2 Tea plantation and other workers

Tea plays an important role in the identity and economy of Sri Lanka. The production of tea in Sri Lanka is still a labour-intensive process as is the case with rubber production. The workforce providing labour on tea and rubber plantations reside in basic dwellings popularly known as "line rooms" provided by the management of the estate. Each estate may have one or more "line rooms" and the residents of these dwellings form a small community. Most workers on the tea plantations are of Indian Tamil origin having been brought to Sri Lanka by the British specifically to work the tea plantations. These groups of labourers tend to skirt the fringes of mainstream Sri Lankan society and services. As opposed to the plight of these people 50 years ago, there have been improvements in their living conditions, rights and the services available to them, including education and health services. The "line room" dwellings for each family are small and as families grow, even extended families tend to live in this limited space, giving rise to a host of socioeconomic issues. The FPA recognized that plantation workers were in need of assistance and support in order to improve their well-being, health and lifestyle. This work was started in the early 1960s. Estates were visited in order to educate the labour force and

> Tea plays an important role in the identity and economy of Sri Lanka. The production of tea in Sri Lanka is still a labour-intensive process as is the case with rubber production

> The FPA also established a hotline to answer any questions on SRH issues. The overwhelming response to the hotline made it clear that more awareness and education on SRH issues was required

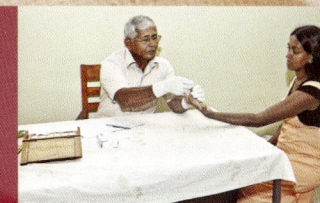

The triumphant journey of FPA Sri Lanka: Sasakawa and beyond: 2004 (Sri Lanka)

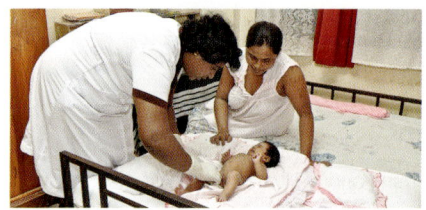
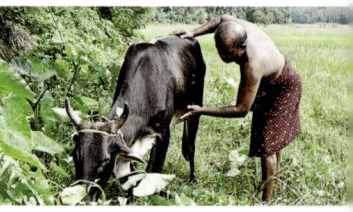

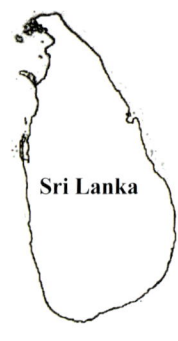

Sri Lanka

Training courses were conducted for estate medical officers and midwives who worked on these estates. As hospitals were sometimes many miles away from the estate, midwives delivered babies

supervisory staff through lectures and film shows on family planning and how it can improve the quality of life. Training courses were also conducted for estate medical officers and midwives who worked on these estates. As hospitals were sometimes many miles away from the estate, midwives delivered babies. With the introduction of these programmes, the FPA witnessed an increased demand by estate populations for contraceptives. In addition to the services provided with the cooperation of the GOSL, a mobile clinic programme was launched in 1971. The mobile clinic could move from estate to estate providing much-needed family planning and support services to pregnant women at their door-step.

Programmes were also conducted for the industrial sector covering men and women employed in factories, and for the various trade unions within the industrial sector. Seminars were conducted with the assistance of the Labour Department and International Labour Organization (ILO). These seminars led to the trade unions considering family planning as an individual right instead of an imposition. Each of these sessions would consist of three talks covering the concept of family planning, the population problem and family planning methods. Short films and slides were also shown on these topics.

7.3   Internally displaced people

In January 2000, the FPA successfully completed an 18-month project to improve the general health and reproductive health status of internally displaced people (IDPs). Funding support for the project was obtained from the IPPF's Netherlands Trust Fund. The displacement of vast numbers of people during the long-drawn-out ethnic conflict in the island led to an unprecedented influx of refugees into makeshift welfare centres in the north-central parts of the country. The IDPs are a vulnerable group who exist on the margins of society with minimal access to basic survival needs and even less by way of SRH facilities. This project was implemented in three north-central districts of the country – Anuradhapura, Polonnaruwa and Puttalam – which had a high concentration of IDPs. At the time of the project, 24 clusters of camps provided shelter for 13 600 families amounting to a refugee population

Sasakawa Health Prize:
STORIES FROM SOUTH-EAST ASIA

of around 69 000. The health and welfare work in each camp was handled by the GOSL with assistance from international and local donor agencies. The bare essentials such as food, clothing and shelter were provided at minimal levels. However, health care remained underserved. The government health-care system did not reach the camps regularly or adequately. In this situation, the health of the IDPs deteriorated rapidly and they proved to be a high-risk group susceptible to communicable diseases. Family planning among couples in the camps was also minimal.

The FPA implemented a project targeting the SRH and basic health needs of the IDPs. The project was implemented in two stages. The first covered a period of 12 months commencing from April 1998 and the second was for a shorter period from August 1999. The primary objective was to improve the health status of the target population and to bring it on a par with that of the national average. The seven specific objectives of the project were: to provide access to quality health/SRH services to the camp community, to improve levels of family planning by one third, to ensure community participation in health/RH awareness creation through trained volunteers and community leaders, to facilitate government health-care services to reach the camp community, to provide SRH information and counselling to adolescents and youth through 48 trained, part-time counsellors, to provide first aid services, and to educate and sensitize the camp community on gender issues.

Maximum community participation ensured the success of this project. The FPA worked through the government agents, rehabilitation officers and religious leaders such as the moulavis of the mosques. A sense of responsibility and ownership of the project was imparted to the community, whose buy-in was necessary, as this was a group of people who had been traumatized by violence and displacement, and fraught with distrust and anxiety. The project was introduced as a high-profile health awareness campaign. During the first few months, the FPA concentrated on general health and sanitation as the camps were in dire need of improved standards of hygiene and cleanliness.

> Programmes were conducted for the industrial sector covering men and women employed in factories, and for the various trade unions within the industrial sector. Seminars were conducted with the assistance of the Labour Department and International Labour Organization (ILO)

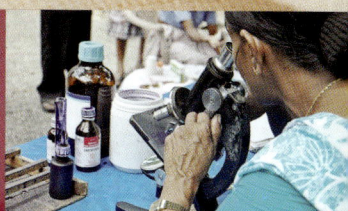

The FPA worked through the government agents, rehabilitation officers and religious leaders such as the moulavis of the mosques

The triumphant journey of FPA Sri Lanka: Sasakawa and beyond: 2004 (Sri Lanka)

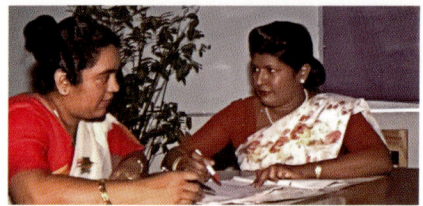
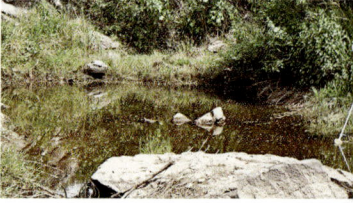

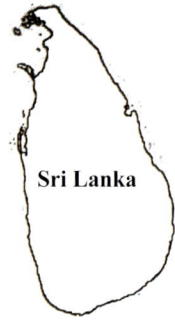
Sri Lanka

The polyclinics proved to be popular and were always well attended. Health-care services to reduce and minimize the prevalence of diseases neglected by the system were offered through 117 polyclinics that served over 34 000 patients

The major problem encountered was language. Most governmental health service providers spoke only Sinhalese and 90% of the IDPs were Muslims and Tamil people who were Tamil speaking. To move beyond the obstacles faced due to language, local doctors, midwives and IDPs were brought together through FPA polyclinics conducted at camp level. Seven different services were delivered simultaneously by the health staff – mother and child health care including contraceptive services, health and education, child dental care, treatment for worms, malaria treatment, general health consultations as well as a pharmaceutical dispensary. The polyclinics proved to be popular and were always well attended. Health-care services to reduce and minimize the prevalence of diseases neglected by the system were offered through 117 polyclinics that served over 34 000 patients.

The project used highly participatory methods to mobilize the camp communities by training 240 young health volunteers – both men and women – living in the camps. During the project they were provided with training, attended seminars and lectures, qualified in first aid (through the offices of the Sri Lanka Red Cross), took part in all the camp's health drives and provided advice on sanitation and hygiene. Intensive awareness drives on HIV/AIDS were carried out by the volunteers. The idea was to create a sense of healing and well-being from within the community, and establish and provide camp-level health committees to provide leadership to the volunteers in carrying out the work. Active volunteers were trained as peer educators to run SRH sessions with young people. They were also encouraged to direct those requiring counselling to the 24 FPA-trained counsellors at the camps. The commitment, enthusiasm and energy of these young volunteers attracted the energy of the media and they were featured on national television and in the print media.

Another challenge was the resistance faced by the predominantly Muslim IDP community. Realizing the patriarchal nature of the community, the FPA reached out to the men of the community through male volunteers to make them understand that contraception meant improved health of the mother and child. Over time, they understood and began to accept the message. For the women in the camps, the project was an eye-opener. Misconceptions were also rife as a result of cultural practices and beliefs. A survey conducted at the beginning of the project in April 1998 showed that 40.6% of the couples within the camps were practising some form of contraception, but only 33% were using modern methods. The project gave them the voice to speak up and discuss their issues with volunteers from among their community.

As a result of this initiative, the government health services began reaching the camps. Public health inspectors started serving the camp communities and, with the assistance of volunteers, found it easier to carry out their work in the camps. The IDPs also started to visit the government facilities for health-care services. The project received the support of the leaders in the camp community. The service support received from the government health-care personnel and the close cooperation and coordination between the GOSL personnel and the FPA was productive and resulted in fruitful completion of the project. The partnership has been cited as an excellent model for cooperation between and among diverse humanitarian agencies.

8. Going online

For sustainability, the FPA maintains an identity that is contemporary. It has added CDs and DVDs with information on SRH issues to the booklets and poster campaigns carried out previously. In the fast-paced age of the internet, the FPA has tapped into cyberspace to extend the services provided and reach out to those in need of support in a manner that ensures privacy, confidentiality and information from a trusted source. The award-winning Happy Life Project made possible with the support of the ICT arm of the GOSL has brought about this innovative approach to handling SRH issues. During the 1960s to the 1990s, the FPA resource centre carried posters to create awareness. However, today with the Happy Life Project, the organization is online to provide support using the latest technology that is available including the world wide web, mobile phones, SMS and e-mail.

Active volunteers were trained as peer educators to run SRH sessions with young people. They were also encouraged to direct those requiring counselling to the 24 FPA-trained counsellors at the camps

Today with the Happy Life Project, the organization is online to provide support using the latest technology that is available including the world wide web, mobile phones, SMS and e-mail

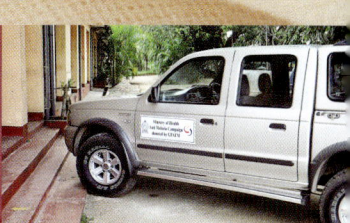

THE TRIUMPHANT JOURNEY OF FPA SRI LANKA: SASAKAWA AND BEYOND: 2004 (SRI LANKA)

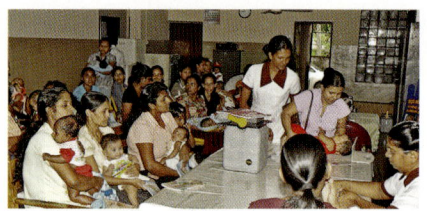
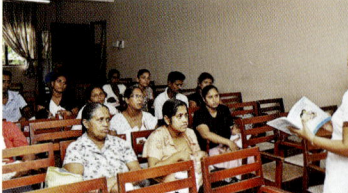

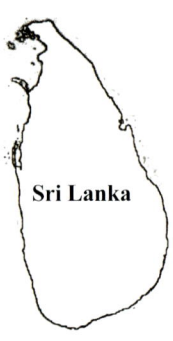

Sri Lanka

Volunteerism has been a part of the organization. This continues till date and the focus is for family planning to be voluntarily accepted by people

9. Using volunteers

Volunteerism has been a part of the organization. This continues till date and the focus is for family planning to be voluntarily accepted by people. On an organizational level, the governance of the FPA is carried out by volunteers who are professionals working towards the empowerment of individuals through the creation of SRH awareness and support systems. From the 1970s, the FPA worked through a system of volunteer committees who would run family planning community projects. Training for volunteers started in areas where family planning community projects were already under way. Volunteers were trained from all over the country including estate medical assistants and midwives. To meet these new training needs, a comprehensive curriculum was drawn up by the FPA based on the early training programmes and the requirements of the volunteers. Local government officers, officers of government departments and officers of the armed forces were trained as peer educators. Voluntary service organizations such as the Rotary Clubs were also trained to conduct family planning programmes for their members. Thus, training activities were broad-based and covered categories such as grass-roots level volunteers, members of community-based organizations, medical personnel, officers belonging to state institutions and members of staff of the FPA.

10. The Sasakawa Award and beyond

Winning the Sasakawa Award in 2004 is testament to the pioneering spirit and commitment of the FPA. In the post-Sasakawa Award era, the FPA has continued to provide the services and support that it is now known and trusted for in Sri Lanka. In order for the work of the FPA to be carried out, it is vital that the organization looks at its survival and sustenance. With a view to ensuring the continuity of the FPA, the organization under its current leadership is working to diversify its donor base and build new partnerships that are mutually beneficial to donor and donee. It is important that future projects undertaken by the FPA be sustainable for the community and the organization.

Sasakawa Health Prize:
STORIES FROM SOUTH-EAST ASIA

During the post-Sasakawa Award period, the importance of proactive thinking and action beyond the sphere of SRH has become clear. Proactive action is a fundamental element of how the FPA provides its services. Today, the FPA works to expand its horizons to include humanitarian services and support. When the devastating tsunami of 2004 struck Sri Lanka, the FPA was not equipped to deal with a natural disaster of this proportion. All action as a result was reactive. The lessons learned from this experience shaped the thinking of the organization in dealing with a humanitarian crisis. During the final 12 months of the ethnic conflict in Sri Lanka, the FPA was ready to provide the humanitarian support required by the IDPs in the northern and eastern parts of the island. The FPA in partnership with the United Nations Population Fund (UNFPA) set up mobile clinics, organized the distribution of hygienic packs and pregnancy kits for women entering their confinement. The FPA also trained individuals as "be-frienders" to focus on listening to the concerns of women. Although this was a new role for the FPA, it was one that provided new opportunities to reach out to groups of society in need of medical and health services, and reproductive health services became a part of the humanitarian assistance provided to IDPs.

10.1 Demographic bonus and increased life expectancy

One third of the current population of 22 million belongs to the workforce due to the stabilized population growth. The lifestyle changes and choices of today have seen an increase in life expectancy among Sri Lankans, especially women. As women become more aware of a sense of autonomy relating to their bodies, they can plan their careers, finances and families to suit their lifestyles and needs. More women in the workforce, in places of power and leadership would bring to the fore gender issues such as discrimination in the workplace and sexual harassment.

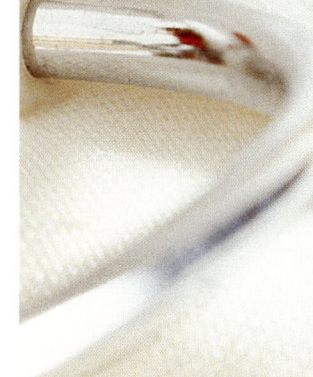

Voluntary service organizations such as the Rotary Clubs were also trained to conduct family planning programmes for their members

The FPA in partnership with the United Nations Population Fund (UNFPA) set up mobile clinics, organized the distribution of hygienic packs and pregnancy kits for women entering their confinement

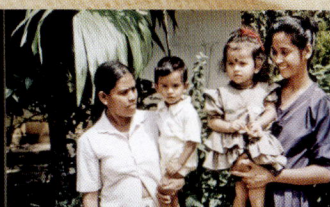

THE TRIUMPHANT JOURNEY OF FPA SRI LANKA: SASAKAWA AND BEYOND: 2004 (SRI LANKA)

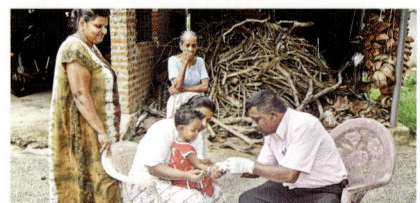
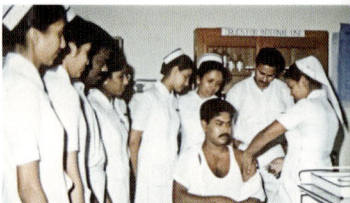

10.2 Meeting the Millennium Development Goals (MDGs)

In keeping with MDG 5 of universal access to SRH by 2015, the FPA works to recognize excluded populations such as those of different sexual orientations. Through its work in SRH care, education, support and counselling, the FPA directly contributes to Universal Access covered by Section 5b of the MDG, and has a major impact on maternal mortality, poverty and AIDS covered under Section 5a of the MDG. Success in this area has been achieved due to the close working relations between the FPA and the Ministry of Health, and relevant departments such as the Family Health Bureau, Health Education Bureau and the National STD/AIDS Control Programme. The FPA works in collaboration with the GOSL at the national, provincial and district levels.

10.3 Moving into the future

Although the sociocultural climate has changed from 1953 to 2010, the spirit of FPA Sri Lanka stays the same as they work to build trust, break new ground, reach out, encourage volunteerism and ensure sustainability for SRH support systems and the organization itself. The story of the FPA is one of "mission accomplished". However, instead of resting on its laurels, the organization firmly believes that with each accomplishment, there are new challenges and goals to work towards. Today, the FPA is of the view that it does not have the luxury of time and the mantra of the organization is to "adapt fast and proactively serve; innovation being the key to survival".

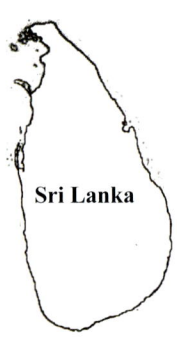

Sri Lanka

Instead of resting on its laurels, the organization firmly believes that with each accomplishment, there are new challenges and goals to work towards

11. Bibliography

1   Department of Census and Statistics, Sri Lanka. http://www.statistics.gov.lk/home.asp - accessed 15 May 2012.

2   De Silva WI. A population projection of Sri Lanka, for the new millennium 2001–2101: trends and implications. Colombo: Institute for Health Policy, 2007.

3   Weerakoon Bradman. Golden jubilee souvenir, 1953–2003. Colombo: Family Planning Association, 2003.

4   Family Planning Association of Sri Lanka.

5   Family Planning Association of Sri Lanka. Annual report (various years). Available at http://www.fpasrilanka.org, Colombo.

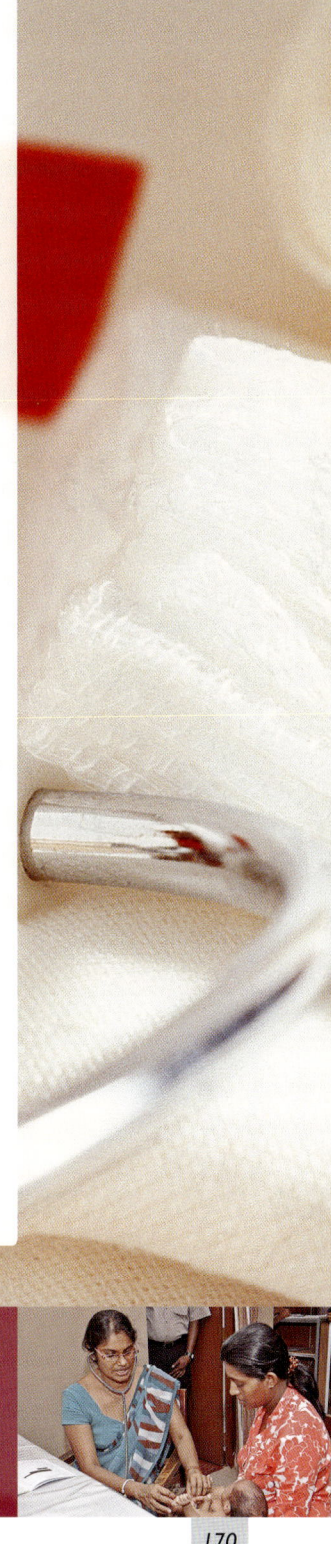

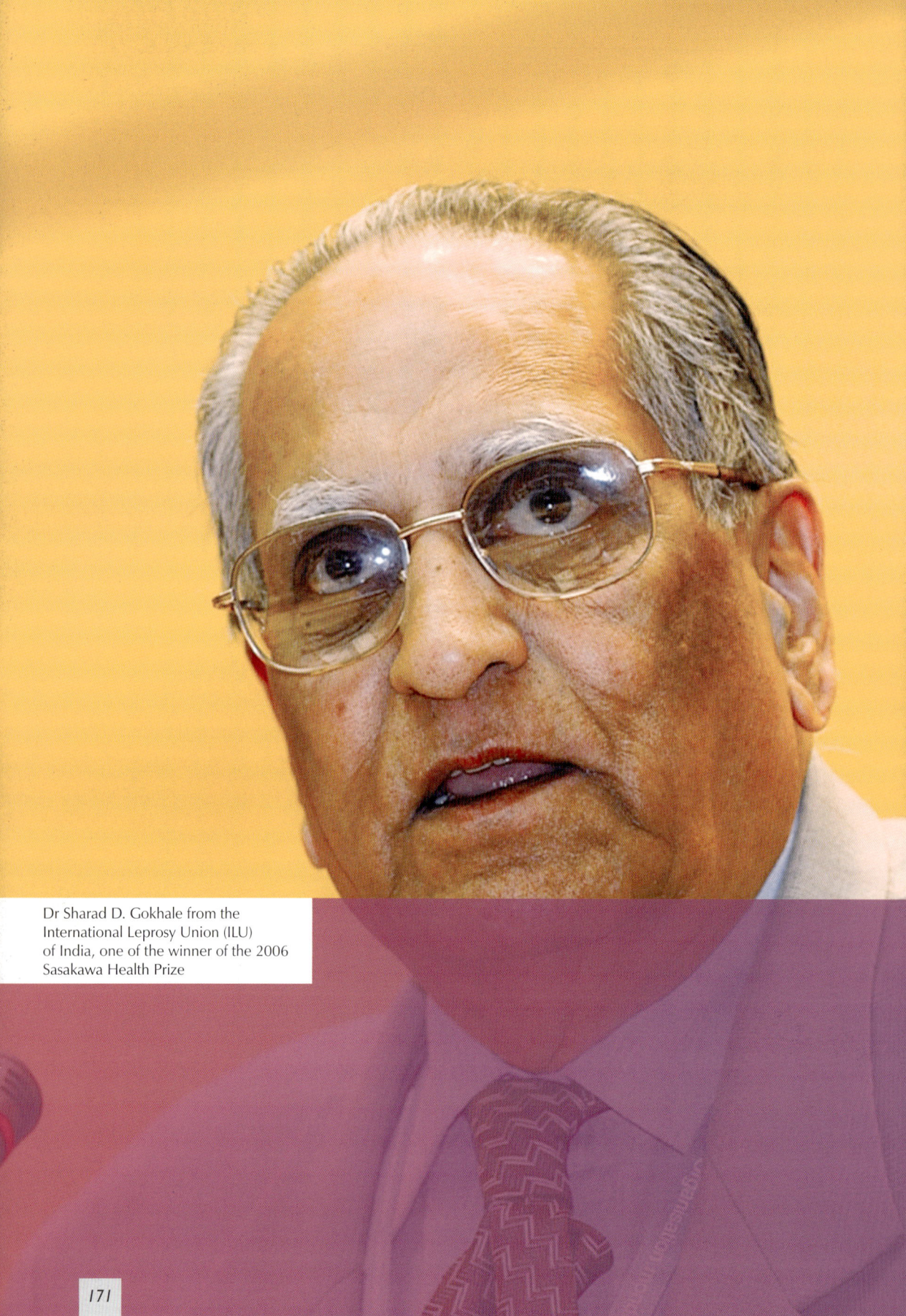

Dr Sharad D. Gokhale from the International Leprosy Union (ILU) of India, one of the winner of the 2006 Sasakawa Health Prize

CHAPTER 11

2006

International Leprosy Union (India): "Life is beautiful"[*]

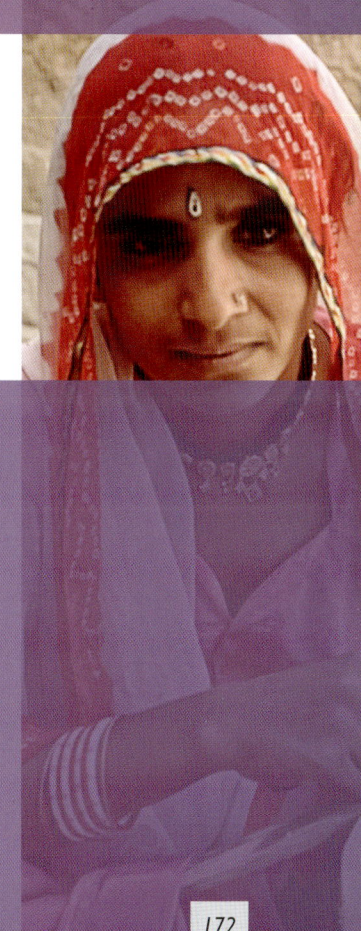

Recipient:
International Leprosy Union
(India)

[*] Initial draft prepared by Dr S.D. Gokhale
International Leprosy Union-Health Alliance,
1779/84, Gurutrayee, Near Bharat Scout Ground,
Sadashiv Peth, Pune-411030, India

ILU was formed with the aim of involving the community in tackling the issue of stigma, social isolation and dehabitation. ILU is an association of Indian nongovernmental organizations (NGOs) with partnership open to NGOs working in other endemic countries

1. Background

Freedom is a natural and basic human aspiration. For centuries, a unique disease called leprosy has succeeded in taking it away from people. People suffering from leprosy have to fight not only against the bacillus Mycobacterium leprae but also against stigma and discrimination, and in gaining dignity as individuals in the community.

The International Leprosy Union (ILU) has taken a position that leprosy is more of a social disease than a medical one. During the late fifties, the development of drugs to treat leprosy was a major achievement in the evolution of this age-old disease. The discovery of multidrug therapy (MDT) in 1981 made it possible for leprosy patients to be cured. At the same time, it became possible to reduce the duration of treatment drastically for some patients – from lifelong treatment to a maximum of two years. As a result, people became less fearful of leprosy and, along with this, the stigma associated with the disease also declined.

In spite of this success in the field of medicine, however, stigma associated with the disease persists and the rights of persons affected by leprosy are still denied in many communities. ILU was formed with the aim of involving the community in tackling the issue of stigma, social isolation and dehabitation. ILU is an association of Indian nongovernmental organizations (NGOs) with partnership open to NGOs working in other endemic countries.

2. The needs of leprosy-affected persons

Leprosy is caused by Mycobacterium leprae, which is a bacillus that attacks the skin and peripheral nerves, and affects parts of the body such as the feet, hands, face and earlobes. Because of the damage to the nerves, the affected person, if left untreated, ultimately develops deformities in the hands, feet and face.

Once leprosy is contracted, immediate treatment with a full course of MDT is of utmost importance. Unfortunately, for those who are diagnosed late, with impairment and disfigurement of the hands, feet and face, it becomes very difficult to reverse these consequences of the disease. For such individuals, care of the damaged eyes, hands and feet becomes an important task for the individual and the health services. Such individuals need support aids and assistive devices. Some of them will require corrective surgery to protect their hands and feet.

Apart from physical aid, the affected person needs psychological help through counselling. The family needs to be told that there is nothing wrong with the person. There should be no fear after the person is cured. Today, there are thousands in India who are completely cured and back with their families, happily occupying respectable positions at work and within their communities.

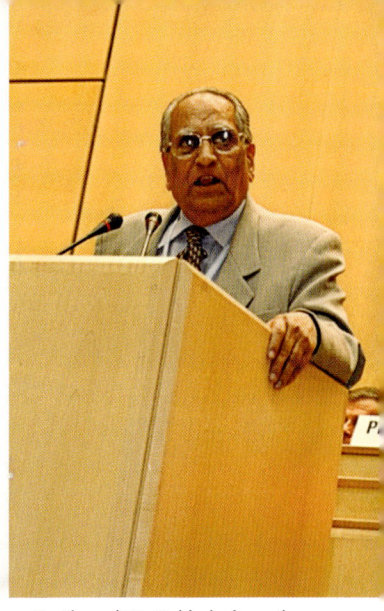

Dr Sharad D. Gokhale from the International Leprosy Union (ILU) of India addressing the 59th World Health Assembly.

Photo credit:
WHO/Peter Williams

3. International Leprosy Union

The International Leprosy Union (ILU) was launched at the regional disability conference on rehabilitation held in Mumbai in 1986. It began with the understanding that leprosy cannot be treated as a medical condition or as a situation where only help in cash or kind can achieve total rehabilitation. It needs efforts from the society to demolish stigma and integrate those affected by leprosy into the general society. This led NGOs from developing countries to form an NGO to deal with issues related to the social and rehabilitation needs of persons affected by leprosy in their own countries. The main activities of ILU are as follows:

- Forum on social issues
- Field work
- Recognition, felicitation and awards
- Research and documentation on human rights issues
- Media and advocacy
- Networking with other organizations

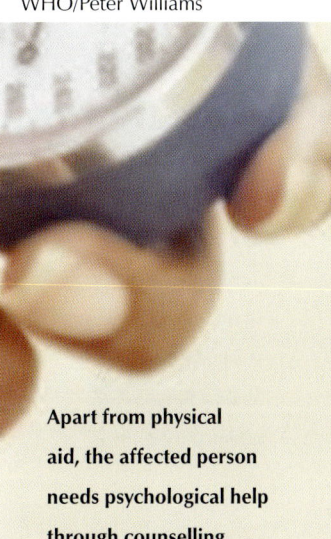

Apart from physical aid, the affected person needs psychological help through counselling. The family needs to be told that there is nothing wrong with the person

The International Leprosy Union (ILU) has taken a position that leprosy is more of a social disease than a medical one. During the late fifties, the development of drugs to treat leprosy was a major achievement in the evolution of this age old disease

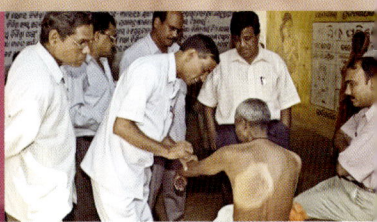

International Leprosy Union (India): "Life is beautiful": 2006 (India)

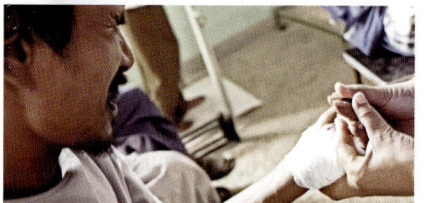 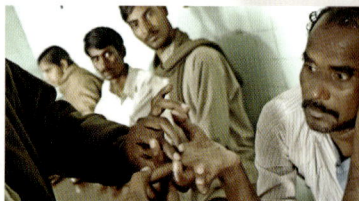

3.1 Forum on social issues

Stigma: ILU approaches the Indian Parliament

Advocacy has been an important issue for ILU. At the International Workshop held at Wardha, India in 1986 by the Gandhi Memorial Leprosy Foundation (GMLF) and ILU, stigma was defined as "a continuum of society's response from total rejection to total acceptance".

ILU joins hands with other organizations on human rights issues associated with leprosy and supports efforts in rectifying existing laws that discriminate against persons affected by leprosy. For example, certain laws in India actually fuel the creation of this stigma. The Indian Lepers Act, 1898 prevented leprosy-affected individuals from travelling on trains, going to public places, etc. A long and arduous battle that lasted for 20 years has helped to remove this law from the statute book. However, dozens of other pieces of legislation exist, which attempt to segregate persons affected by leprosy from mainstream society. Consider, for instance, the Juvenile Justice Act, 1986, which states that if a child is suffering from leprosy one must segregate and put the child into a leprosy home. Another case is the Prevention of Begging Act, 1959. There are 16 such laws that create stigmatization. This is grossly wrong and is currently seen to be unnecessary.

There is a dire need to change these laws and modify government policies because they effectively take away the basic human rights of affected persons. The Prevention of Begging Act, 1959 in Bombay mentions that a leprosy-affected person has to be committed to a leprosy institution indefinitely till death. The point is: do we have the right to infringe upon the liberty of a person in such a manner? Also, the Hindu Marriage Act, 1955 and the Muslim Marriage Act, 1955 need to be amended, as they allow divorce on the grounds of leprosy.

> **ILU joins hands with other organizations on human rights issues associated with leprosy and supports efforts in rectifying existing laws that discriminate against persons affected by leprosy**

Sasakawa Health Prize:
STORIES FROM SOUTH-EAST ASIA

National consultations

Consultations were held in Raipur, Chattisgarh in January 2004 and in New Delhi in June 2004 on "Advocacy strategies and the role of the media in elimination of leprosy in high-endemic states". State- and district-level consultations were also held in Pune, Maharashtra State in June 2004; Patna, Bihar State in August 2004; Bhubaneshwar, Orissa State in December 2004; Lucknow, Uttar Pradesh State in December 2004; Kolkata, West Bengal State in May 2005; and Ranchi, Jharkand State in November 2005.

Workshop

A workshop was also jointly organized with WHO in May 2005 in Pune on "Issues surrounding families and children living in the shadow of leprosy and HIV/AIDS".

Collaboration with the Gandhi Memorial Leprosy Foundation

ILU collaborates closely with the GMLF in organizing meetings and seminars. It works jointly with the GMLF in advocating for changes in the existing laws that discriminate against persons affected by leprosy. It provides help in conducting the selection process for the International Gandhi Award that is given annually to outstanding workers and organizations in the field of leprosy from all over the world.

3.2 Field work

From rejection to self-care

As far as patients are concerned, those who are under treatment or even those who have been cured are not accepted back in society. They are abandoned by their families and rejected by their village folk. ILU's task is to change the psyche of the community and that of the media, as it reaches the community at large.

> ILU's task is to change the psyche of the community and that of the media, as it reaches the community at large

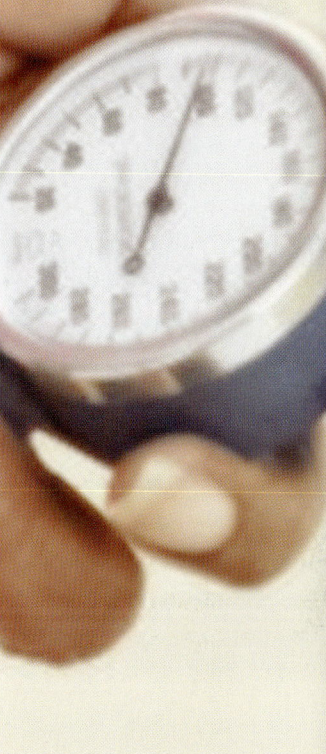

Group photo - Dr Sharad D. Gokhale from the International Leprosy Union of India (far right).

Photo credit: WHO/Peter Williams

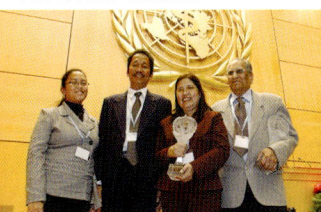

> The Prevention of Begging Act, 1959 in Bombay mentions that a leprosy affected person has to be committed to a leprosy institution indefinitely till death

International Leprosy Union (India): "Life is beautiful": 2006 (India)

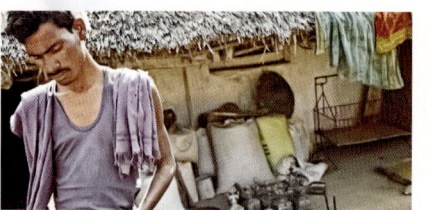 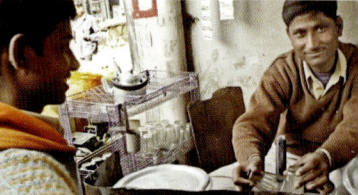

ILU started developing programmes that begin with self-care. Self-care implies teaching a patient how to take care of their feet and hands. By supporting such initiatives, persons affected by leprosy are able to prevent new disabilities from developing or existing ones from getting worse. It also helps persons affected by leprosy to obtain certain appliances such as proper footwear, wheelchairs and crutches, which allow them to lead a productive life in society.

Looking after children and family members

ILU sponsors children and family members who have to live under the shadow of leprosy and HIV/AIDS. Support for education is provided to children on a yearly basis. The core belief of ILU is that sponsoring children of persons affected by leprosy will allow them to live with their own families rather than in institutions. This effort has been successful since 1995. It also provides the next generation with developmental opportunities that will help them improve their lives in future.

True rehabilitation: factory run by persons affected by leprosy in Pune

With support from industrialists, ILU was able to set up a machine shop to produce automobile parts for Tata Engineering and Locomotive Company (TELCO). The TELCO trucks have a locking system that is fairly complicated. It is now made in the workshop staffed by persons affected by leprosy. The factory is unique in the sense that it is a cooperative run by persons affected by leprosy. These individuals take all the decisions with regard to production, financial policies, employment, or sharing profits among themselves. This initiative has been internationally recognized and has received the ILU award.

Providing small loans

Small loans are provided to persons affected by leprosy so that they are able to become productive members of society as well as their families. This allows them to be independent and empowers them to make decisions with regard to their daily lives and interaction with members of the community.

3.3 Recognition, felicitation and awards

Lokdoots and Madhyamdoots: the historic concepts

Apart from the mainstream media, it is vital to get individuals who have been cured on a public platform so that they can tell their stories. This "first person" experience sharing is certainly more credible than any other form of advocacy. A man who has suffered can tell his tale with great confidence. When he says, "Look, I had leprosy, but I am happy, I am cured. I am working; I am married and have a family." ILU has been supporting persons affected by leprosy (called Lokdoots, meaning peoples' messengers), to spread awareness about leprosy elimination and prevention of stigma. In the endemic states of India, ILU registers persons who have been cured of leprosy as volunteers.

In addition, there are thousands of Boy Scouts and Girl Guides who are working as volunteers in this field. A large number of mediapersons from the electronic, print and online media have agreed to become Madhyamdoots (media messengers) to generate awareness about leprosy, work towards the elimination of stigma and aid in rehabilitating persons affected by leprosy into society.

ILU has been following this pattern, which started when a number of cured individuals were publicly felicitated by the former President of India, Sri R. Venkatraman and the WHO Goodwill Ambassador, Yohei Sasakawa. This recognition provided them with confidence and supported them in their journey back to the society where they once belonged. As a part of his speech during the felicitation ceremony, one of the Lokdoots said, "My friends, if society does not come to you, let us go to the society and tell them that there is nothing wrong with us."

The struggle of persons affected by leprosy and its positive coverage in the mainstream media will help reduce the stigma that has been prevalent for ages. Society will have to listen to the changes occurring in leprosy and rectify its response in an inclusive and non-stigmatizing way.

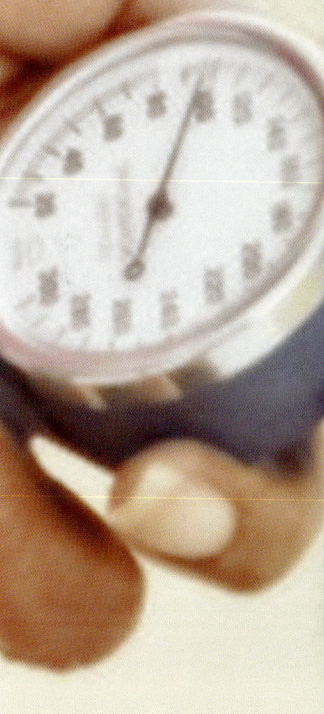

ILU sponsors children and family members who have to live under the shadow of leprosy and HIV/AIDS

> The struggle of persons affected by leprosy and its positive coverage in the mainstream media will help reduce the stigma that has been prevalent for ages

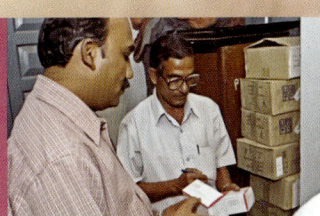

INTERNATIONAL LEPROSY
UNION (INDIA): "LIFE IS
BEAUTIFUL": 2006 (INDIA)

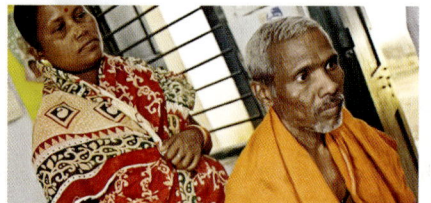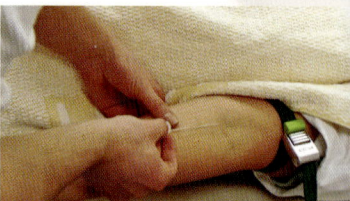

Award for outstanding work in leprosy

Each year, ILU gives an award to outstanding individuals and organizations for the work done in uplifting the lives of persons affected by leprosy.

3.4 Media and advocacy

Fighting the stigma: media fellowships (Madhyamdoot)

The next significant question that arises in this battle is: how do we change the mindset of society and use the media in this process? ILU has started a fellowship programme for media people to fund their visits to the homes of leprosy-affected persons who have been cured. They can talk to the family members and write about their experiences. With awareness generated on the issue, it will be easier for the community to accept such persons. In the battle against the stigma attached to leprosy, ILU organized media partnership workshops in eight cities of India in late 2005, reaching out to around 250 development and health journalists across all major media houses in the country.

Apart from the media fellowship programme, ILU's aim is to counsel families living under the shadow of leprosy. Rehabilitation means making a leprosy-affected person economically self-sufficient, socially accepted and psychologically confident. Rehabilitation International and WHO convened a workshop in Geneva where a representative of ILU was invited. At this meeting, a standard definition was evolved.

Media workshops

A media workshop was held in New Delhi in January 2005 in collaboration with the Centre for Media Research. Eight media partnership workshops were also held to sensitize over 300 media personnel across India to seek their support in getting across the right message about leprosy in their coverage.

Each year, ILU gives an award to outstanding individuals and organizations for the work done in uplifting the lives of persons affected by leprosy

179

Production of educational materials

A quarterly newsletter called the Last Mile was started in January 2005 and is published every quarter. The newsletter covers the outstanding work of the Lokdoots and honours the efforts they make at the community level. ILU has published the following books:

- *Dignity regained*, 2005, published by Icons media
- *Human face of leprosy*, 1998, published by Ameya Prakashan
- *Dehabilitation intervention strategies*, 1993, published by Somaiya Publications, and
- *Rehabilitation policies and programmes*, 1984, published by Somaiya Publications

A film titled "Chalo Lokdoot Bane" (let us become the messengers of the people) was produced and screened in January 2005. ILU also collaborated with the BBC World Trust to produce a film on reducing stigma and discrimination in India and Nepal.

A campaign was started in 2005 by congratulating persons affected by leprosy for their successful treatment and being able to lead a normal life in society. Posters were designed with photographs of individuals from various fields of work – one was a manager, the other a nurse and another a doctor. The title of the poster was, "There is one thing common amongst us" and in very fine print below, it stated, "We were all leprosy patients."

3.5 Research and documentation on human right issues

The United Nations Human Rights Commission has established a subcommission on this subject, which made a trip to Pune, India in March 2005. ILU helped in organizing a workshop on human rights. ILU was also requested to conduct a survey and collect data on the subject of stigma and human rights. The Indian Human Rights Commission also requested ILU to carry out surveys to collect such data.

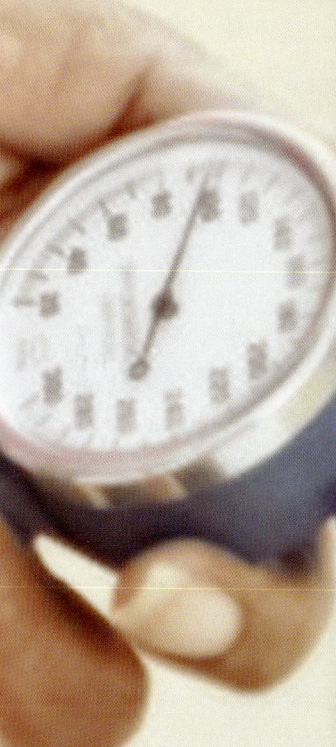

ILU's aim is to counsel families living under the shadow of leprosy. Rehabilitation means making a leprosy-affected person economically self-sufficient, socially accepted and psychologically confident

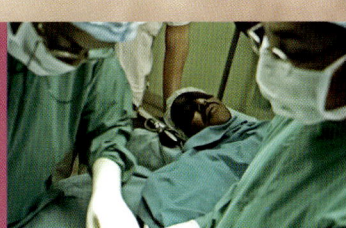

ILU also collaborated with the BBC World Trust to produce a film on reducing stigma and discrimination in India and Nepal

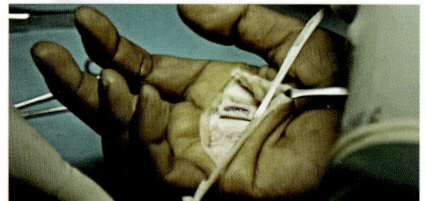
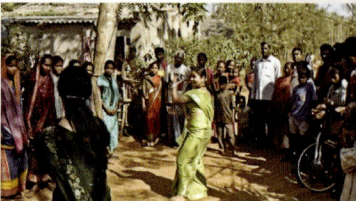

ILU took the initiative to develop a grievance redress cell. It collects complaints on breaches of human rights. ILU examines them and forwards them to the State and National Human Rights Commission, which examine the complaints and re-establish the rights.

3.6 Networking with other organizations

ILU has been successful in networking with the International Leprosy Association (ILA) and International Association for Integration, Dignity and Economic Advancement (IDEA) in promoting the rights of persons affected by leprosy, by participating in the various meetings and forums held by them. It continues to also network with various media organizations throughout India to get support from the media in sending out positive information about the disease as well as about the rights of persons affected by leprosy.

The discovery of multidrug therapy (MDT) in 1981 made it possible for leprosy patients to be cured

Sasakawa Health Prize:
STORIES FROM SOUTH-EAST ASIA

4. Conclusion

Through its programmes, ILU hopes to instil self-confidence and empower persons affected by leprosy. It also hopes to generate awareness of self-care along with the provision of development opportunities for economic rehabilitation. Through these efforts, it hopes that the disease will become part of history and that India will achieve Mahatma Gandhi's dream of becoming a leprosy-free country.

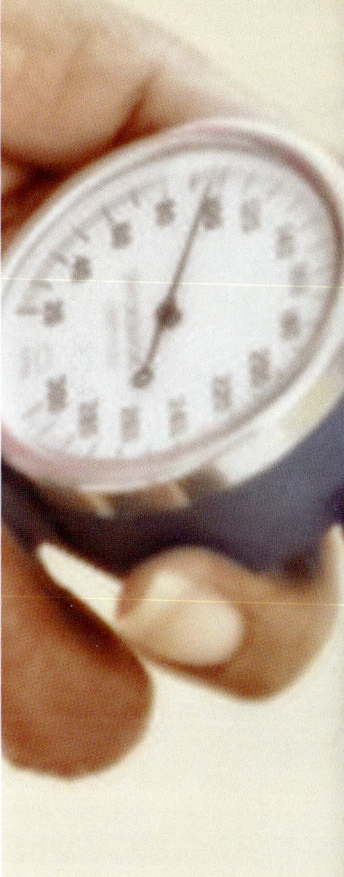
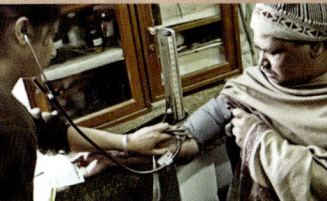

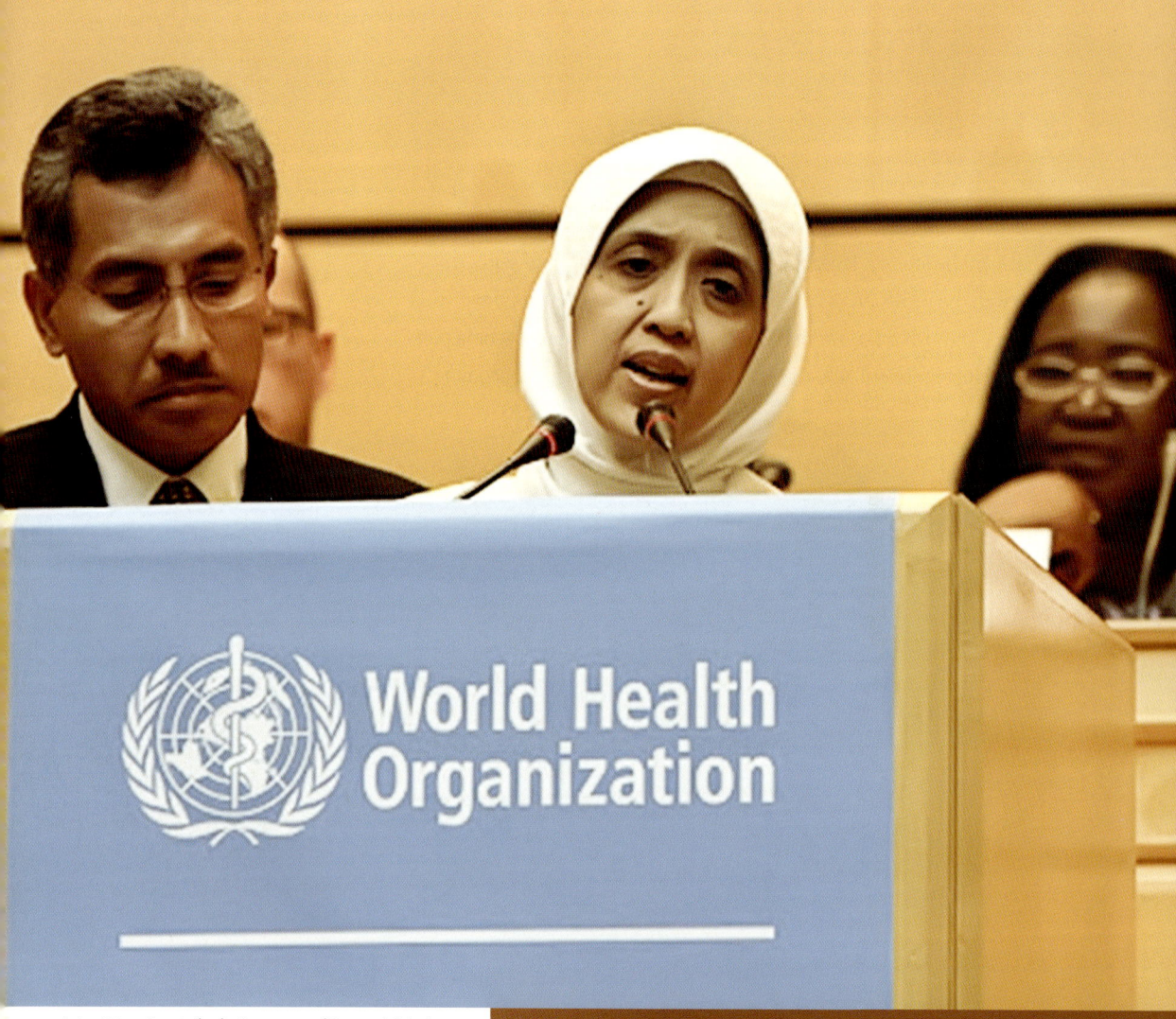

Mrs Dian Syarief, chairperson of Syamsi Dhuha Foundation (SDF), winner of the Sasakawa Health Prize, addressing the 65th World Health Assembly on behalf of her foundation

CHAPTER 12

2006

Never give up [*]

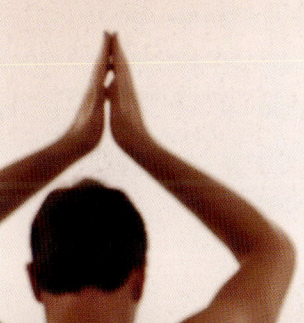

Recipient:
Syamsi Dhuha Foundation
(Indonesia)

---
[*] Syamsi Dhuha Foudation (SDF)
Jl. Ir. H. Juanda 369 Komp. DDK No. 1
Bandung 40135 – Indonesia

S yamsi Dhuha, which means morning light, was born out of gratitude for God's unfathomable love and grace, which shines through a "disaster" of an ailment

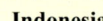

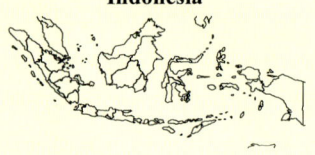

1. Introduction

The Syamsi Dhuha Foundation (SDF) is located in Bandung, Indonesia. Syamsi Dhuha, which means morning light, was born out of gratitude for God's unfathomable love and grace, which shines through a "disaster" of an ailment. An ailment is often perceived as a tragedy, but it can also morph into an extraordinary expression of God's love and grace.

Few people know about the disease named lupus, or systemic lupus erythematosus (SLE), which is a chronic autoimmune disease. It is also known as the "great imitator", as it can mimic the symptoms of various other diseases, causing difficulty in diagnosis. Its cause and cure are unknown. If it is not detected early and treated appropriately, its consequences can be as fatal as those of cancer. It can attack various bodily systems and organs. The symptoms range from mild to serious, and could be even life-threatening. Some factors suspected of triggering lupus include genetic predisposition, hormones and the environment (medicine, poison, food and sunlight). Lupus patients undergo a dramatic change in their personal and family lives, which is occasionally very hard to cope with. To some, their direct involvement with this ailment, either as a patient or supporter, has been an experience that should be patients, doctors, nurses, hospitals and a wider public.

2. The beginning

SDF began by realizing the value of this experience. Initially SDF, through one of its programmes, "Care for lupus", sought to encourage the friends of odapus (people living with lupus) and their families, through various activities that benefit communities beyond the lupus circle. In line with its mission ("as an avenue of charity to attain joy in this world and beyond the earthly life"), SDF aspires to involve everyone, not just odapus, in many activities that can benefit individuals and others.

Few people know about the disease named lupus, or systemic lupus erythematosus (SLE), which is a chronic autoimmune disease

Sasakawa Health Prize:
STORIES FROM SOUTH-EAST ASIA

With approximately 200 000 people living with lupus or 0.1% of the country's total population, Indonesian lupus peer groups are expected to not only provide education and advocacy to help lupus patients, but are also required to find ways to lessen the financial and mental burden. Currently, there are very few peer groups in Indonesia; one of them is SDF and the other is the Jakarta-based Yayasan Lupus Indonesia (Indonesian Lupus Foundation).

Learning from how peer groups operate in other countries, SDF has been began conducting activities to help and support lupus patients and build public awareness about lupus since 2004. Starting with just 10 members, SDF's membership has grown to almost 600 members currently. The first step taken by the Foundation was to collect information to establish a database that would help create a better picture of the demography of patients. The database, though a modest is the primary source of identifying what needs to be done to support them. Through this database, SDF encourages university students from several disciplines to undertake theses on lupus.

One of major challenges facing lupus patients in Indonesia is the fact that many of them have financial difficulties due to the relatively high cost of medication, and most of them are not covered by private health insurance. This directed SDF's priority objective of lessening the financial burden by building networks with clinical laboratories and pharmacists to provide discounts for lupus patients. Supported by the Indonesian Rheumatism Association (IRA), SDF approached the Ministry of Health to provide low-cost or free drugs for lupus patients, as provided for AIDS patients.

SDF lobbies with the media and others to support awareness campaigns and public education through seminars and talk shows to generate publicity about the disease. A unique approach is to strengthen the spiritual aspects of patients. In a support session called Contemplation, lupus patients are assisted to strengthen their faith by cultivating a belief

SDF aspires to involve everyone, not just odapus, in many activities that can benefit individuals and others

One of major challenges facing lupus patients in Indonesia is the fact that many of them have financial difficulties due to the relatively high cost of medication

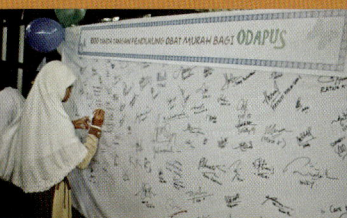

Syamsi Dhuha Foundation, Indonesia

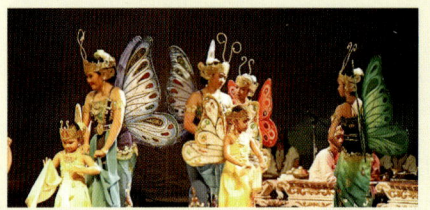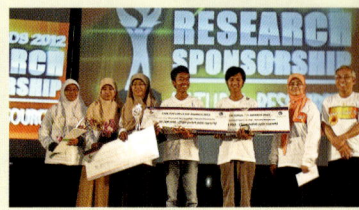

Indonesia

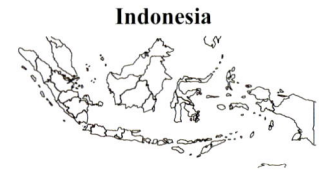

The Foundation focuses on education and socialization programme, and the Care for lupus

that suffering from a sickness is not the end of the world. In other words, no matter how bad the physical condition, the soul and mind need to be peaceful and healthy. Making friends with lupus instead of fighting against it is a unique approach introduced by SDF to cope with lupus. An article on this subject was written by Ms Dian Syarief, the founder and chairperson of SDF and herself a victim of lupus, and published in the local newspaper, Jakarta Post.

Despite very limited resources, including finances, human capital, technology and public support, SDF continues working with many parties, striving to face the challenges and hoping to be a role model for other peer groups in Indonesia.

3. Activities at the Syamsi Dhuha Foundation

The Foundation focuses on three major activities under the "Care for lupus and care for low vision" programme. These aim to improve the quality of life of people living with lupus and low vision. They include a support group programme, an education and socialization programme, and the Care for lupus SDF awards.

3.1 Support group programme

Under the support group programme, which is supported by many volunteers including doctors, SDF provides information to patients and their families about lupus and low vision by answering questions raised by them. Text (SMS), e-mail, phone and other communication channels, including the social media, are used to communicate with members and the public at large. Under this programme, some regular activities are also carried out, such as sharing sessions and contemplation, sports and recreational activities, and an English conversation club. Besides lupus, the Foundation also has an empowering programme to help improve the quality of life of people with low vision. Some programmes that have been conducted include the Shiatsu Massage Training and Certification Programme, Computer Training and Certification Programme for low vision and blind people, and writing skills for low vision and blind people.

3.2 Education and socialization programme

Realizing that lupus is still a relatively unknown disease and the difficulties doctors have in diagnosing it, the education and socialization programme is an important aspect of the Foundation's activities. The target audiences for this education and socialization programme are not only patients and their families, but also medical doctors and the media. Primary care doctors, as first-line health providers, have to be aware of the symptoms and know how to arrive at a diagnosis of lupus. Therefore, the Foundation has initiated training for medical doctors to help them perform their tasks in rural areas. With the cooperation of the local government, two training sessions for primary care doctors in rural areas have been held, and were attended by more than 200 participants. Besides providing training to patients and medical professionals, SDF held lupus training for the media in 2011, as the media plays an important role in bringing awareness of lupus to the public at large.

Under the education and socialization programme, SDF has published some books and one music album:

- Miracle of love, journeying with lupus towards God (2008)
- Love enables me to raise up (2009)
- Care for lupus (music album, 2009)
- Luppy my cheeky friend (animation book and DVD about lupus, 2010)
- The cheeky Luppy is here again (questions and answers on lupus, 2011)
- Luppy's note, the medical diary (2012)

To make it easier to explain lupus, SDF created an animated character named "Luppy". In addition to books, SDF has published articles in the media, and submitted a poster presentation to the International Congress on Lupus, in Shanghai, China in 2007 and in Vancouver, Canada in 2010. This effort has increased awareness of lupus and the existence of the Foundation, both locally and internationally. Three abstracts and poster presentations were submitted to the

> The target audiences for this education and socialization programme are not only patients and their families, but also medical doctors and the media

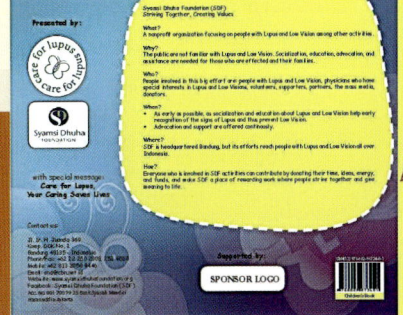
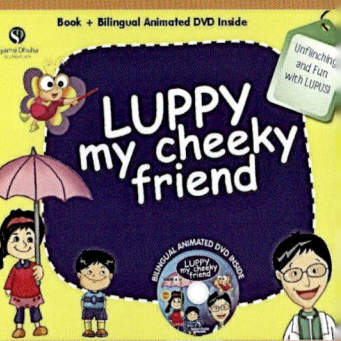

Syamsi Dhuha Foundation, Indonesia

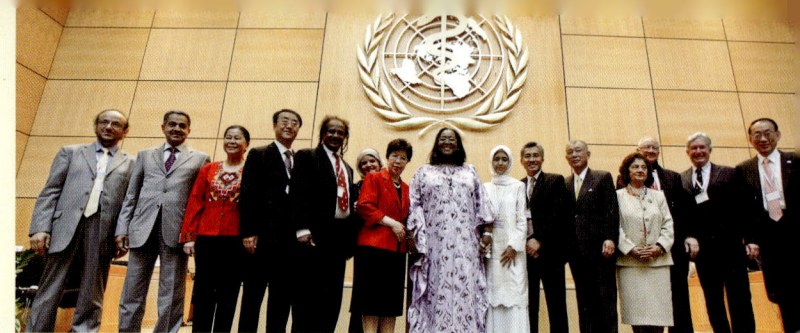

Award winners and representatives of the foundations presenting awards are applauded by assembled delegates

Indonesia

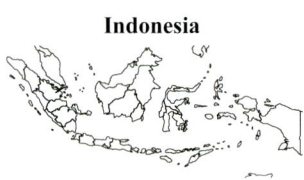

As part of the global lupus community, SDF actively promotes awareness of lupus

8th and 9th International Congress on SLE in Shanghai and Vancouver, respectively:

- Strengthening the faith – a spiritual healing for lupus patients
- Challenges for Indonesian's lupus peer group
- How to make friends with lupus

During the 9th International Congress on SLE in Vancouver, SDF was invited as one of the four panelists to speak at the Global Voluntary Initiative Discussion, together with representatives from the Lupus Foundation of Canada, Lupus Europe and Lupus Foundation of America. SDF was among the 29 recipients of the "International Lifetime Achievement Award" from the Committee of the Congress.

As part of the global lupus community, SDF actively promotes awareness of lupus. It is increasingly drawing the government's attention to the disease by conducting an annual event to commemorate World Lupus Day (WLD). The WLD annual gathering is one example of promoting awareness, educating patients and the public, as well as creating an understanding of what lupus is and how to live with it. This WLD annual event has become a forum for almost all stakeholders: doctors, nurses, patients, hospitals, pharmaceutical companies, government officers, universities, students, volunteers and the media. The agenda includes free consultation for lupus patients and the public with many specialist doctors, Walk for Lupus, volunteers on the street, lupus talk show and seminar, bazaar and exhibition, and an art and music performance. This event has proven successful in raising the motivation of those with lupus and serves as an excellent media event to raise awareness, caring and cooperation among stakeholders.

As a result of the initial WLD gatherings in 2004 and 2006, SDF realized the difficulties of many poor people in accessing major lupus drugs. After a discussion with and support from the Indonesian Association of

Rheumatology, SDF initiated a meeting with the Minister of Health in 2006 to advocate for the distribution of low-cost lupus drugs and to include lupus drugs in the eligible drugs list within the national health insurance programme for poor people (jamkesnas). During the meeting, a petition signed by 1500 people was delivered to the Ministry of Health. In 2012, the foundation also proposed initiating a programme called "Special channel for lupus drugs distribution" to the Ministry of Health to overcome the imbalance and inequity in distribution of lupus drugs, especially to the villages, and rural and remote areas.

3.3 Care for lupus SDF awards

In 2011, SDF initiated the "Care for lupus SDF awards". Three categories of awards were created – research sponsorships award, writing competition award and lifetime achievement award. SDF strives to hold this programme on an annual basis. The objectives of this programme are:

- To strengthen and enhance cooperation among relevant parties in Indonesia for the control of lupus
- To encourage and support research on finding supplementary therapies and herbal-based medicines for lupus
- To increase national awareness of and caring for people with lupus
- To appreciate local institutions, health professionals, patients and the public at large who by word, deed, example or act have advanced local efforts to understand, treat, and/or prevent SLE and its consequences.

In 2012, in addition to the research sponsorship for herbal supplements, one category of research was added, i.e. "All about lupus" to improve the quality of life of people living with lupus. Thirty-five research proposals were submitted (increased from 15 in 2011) from several universities in Indonesia.

> The foundation also proposed initiating a programme called "Special channel for lupus drugs distribution" to the Ministry of Health to overcome the imbalance and inequity in distribution of lupus drugs

One of major challenges facing lupus patients in Indonesia is the fact that many of them have financial difficulties due to the relatively high cost of medication

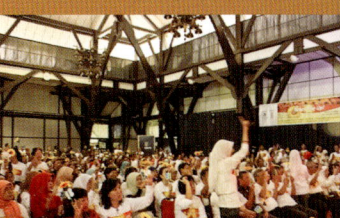

SYAMSI DHUHA
FOUNDATION, INDONESIA

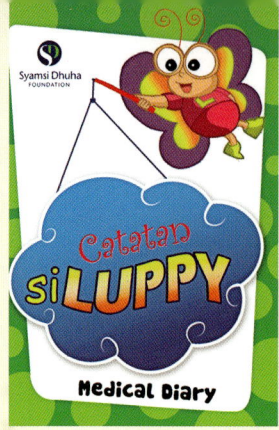
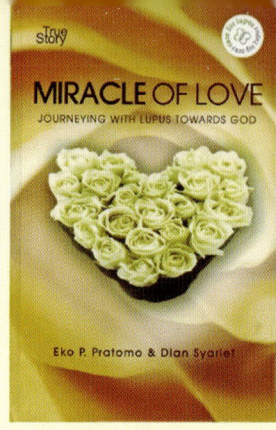

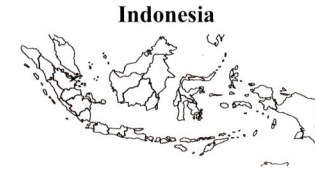

Indonesia

SDF aims to have a comprehensive lupus clinic, where various specialist doctors will attend, and diagnostics and rehabilitation are integrated in one place

The judges consisted of professors, lecturers and medical doctors from the School of Pharmacy, Institute of Technology, Bandung and Faculty of Medicine, Padjadjaran University. They selected three winners from among 26 proposals for herbal supplements, and two winners from among nine proposals for "All about lupus". The award, IDR 30 million (US$ 3100), was granted to the respective winners to defray research expenses. The natural resources being studied are jackfruit seed, sweet potato and Kalanchoe pinnata.

Ten articles on the topic of lupus published in the media were submitted for the writing competition this year and three of them were selected as winners.

In the lifetime achievement category, the committee selected 10 individuals, doctors and institutions for their work in supporting people with lupus and their families, promoting public education and awareness about lupus, and striving for a call to action by the government to increase financial support for lupus research, awareness and patient services.

In the long run, SDF aims to have a comprehensive lupus clinic, where various specialist doctors will attend, and diagnostics and rehabilitation are integrated in one place.

4. Conclusion

During the introductory speech before the Award presentation, Mr Yohei Sasakawa of the Sasakawa Memorial Health Foundation stated that besides the innovative work done by the Foundation, what was even more interesting was that the work was initiated and led by a lupus patient with low vision. Ms Dian Syarief, chairperson of SDF, was diagnosed with lupus in 1999. She had to undergo several major surgeries: six craniotomies due to brain abscess, gallbladder removal, uterus removal, among others. She also suffers from low vision, as she had lost 95% of her eyesight due to brain abscess. Despite struggling with her own illness, her desire to spread awareness about the disease and help others was instrumental in motivating and mobilizing others to get involved and work together with her to run the Foundation.

"Care for lupus, your caring save lives"; "Low vision, care and share" and "NEVER GIVE UP!" are the three messages she always conveys in motivating her lupus and low vision friends and others.

5. Epilogue

Goodwill for Indonesia was evident at the Palais de Nations in Geneva on 24 May 2012 when the Syamsi Dhuha Foundation (SDF) was awarded the Sasakawa Health Prize 2012 by the President of the Sixty-fifth World Health Assembly, Professor Therese N'Dri Yoman. The Director-General of the World Health Organization (WHO) Dr Margaret Chan and Mr Yohei Sasakawa were also present. The SDF received the award for its ongoing commitment to various innovations and activities that have increased the government's and community's awareness of the management of lupus in Indonesia. Delegates from WHO Member States attending the award ceremony were moved when the Founder and Chairperson of the Foundation, Ms Dian Syarief, made an acceptance speech in English. In her address, Ms Syarief thanked the Sasakawa Foundation and WHO for their appreciation of the efforts conducted in Indonesia.

Mr Eko Pratomo, the founder of SDF, expressed his gratitude at having received the award and said that it was shared with everyone who had worked hard shoulder-to-shoulder with SDF in running various education, socialization, support and research programmes to improve the quality of life for lupus and low vision patients ever since SDF was born eight years ago.

The honourable achievements of Dian and Eko through their Foundation have helped Indonesia's humanitarian diplomatic initiatives in an international forum.

> The SDF received the award for its ongoing commitment to various innovations and activities that have increased the government's and community's awareness of the management of lupus in Indonesia

> Mr Eko Pratomo, the founder of SDF, expressed his gratitude at having received the award and said that it was shared with everyone who had worked hard shoulder-to-shoulder with SDF

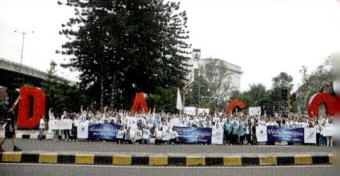

SYAMSI DHUHA
FOUNDATION, INDONESIA

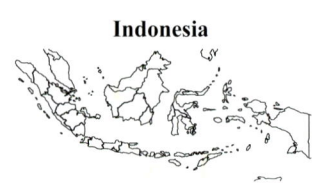
Indonesia

> Limitations are a part of life, and they exist in every country in the world. What we can do is to keep alive our zeal to survive and to thrive, and our effort to reach the goals

Ms Dian Syarief's acceptance speech at the 65th World Health Assembly, 2012

Distinguished Delegates, Ladies and Gentlemen,

We thank the Sasakawa Foundation and the World Health Organization for their appreciation of our endeavour in Indonesia.

For us, being part of millions of people worldwide who have lost their prime health and eyesight, life has taught us amazing lessons. Indeed, having good health and being able to see are two indispensable, invaluable aspects of life. They cannot be substituted with anything else. We didn't realize this truth when we still had them and took them for granted.

Limitations are a part of life, and they exist in every country in the world. What we can do is to keep alive our zeal to survive and to thrive, and our effort to reach the goals. Even if we have to lose to a disease, we shall concede defeat with honour because we will have done our best with all of our strength.

As Hilary Rodham Clinton said once: "I can accept losing. I cannot accept quitting."

Every gesture, every action of care from one person to another will be a source of encouragement and power to survive together in doing our best.

Never give up! Care for lupus; your caring saves lives.

Sasakawa Health Prize:
STORIES FROM SOUTH-EAST ASIA

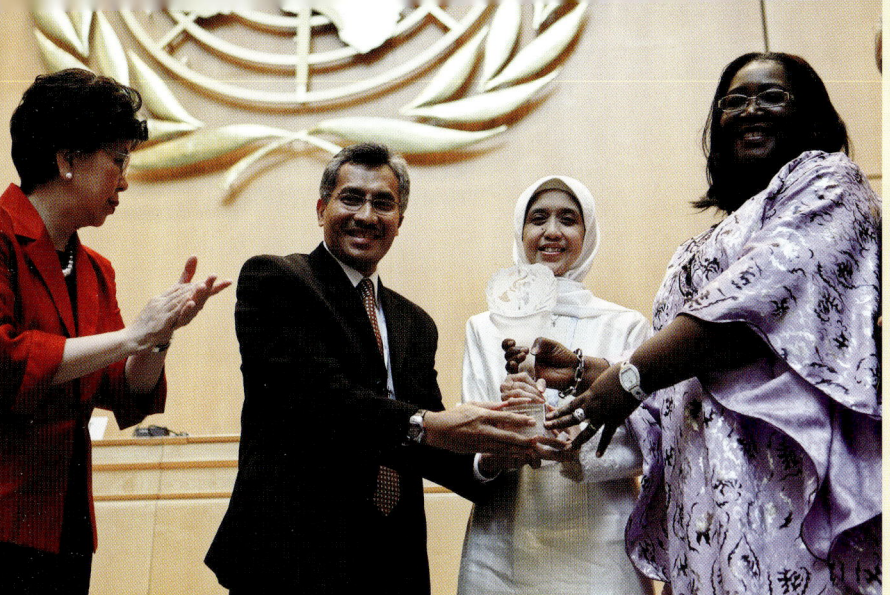

Professor Thérèse N'Dri-Yoman, President of the 65th World Health Assembly, presents Mrs Dian Syarief and Mr Eko Pratomo with the 2012 Sasakawa Health Prize as the WHO Director-General, Dr Margaret Chan, applauds

Care for Lupus
Music Album

Song List
1. Care for lupus
2. Light up the world with the ray of our heart
3. Cintamu (Theme song "Miracle of Love")
4. Sahabat setia
5. Tiada waktu tersisa
6. Kau tak sendiri
7. Detik hidup
8. Victory within me

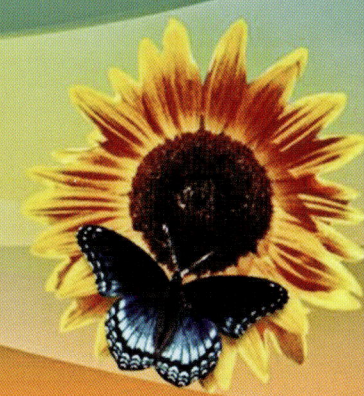

 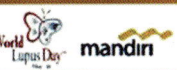 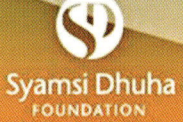

Syamsi Dhuha
FOUNDATION

Annex 1

Statutes of the Sasakawa Health Prize
(as amended in January 1998)

Article 1
Establishment

Under the title of the "Sasakawa Health Prize", a Prize is established within the framework of the World Health Organization, which shall be governed by the following provisions.

Article 2
The Founder

The Prize is established upon the initiative of and with funds provided by Mr Ryoichi Sasakawa, Chairman of the Japan Shipbuilding Industry Foundation and President of the Sasakawa Memorial Health Foundation.

Article 3
Capital

The Founder endows the Prize with an initial capital in Japan of US$ 1 million. The capital of the Prize may be increased by income from its undistributed reserves or by gifts and bequests. The Founder shall designate the Sasakawa Memorial Health Foundation to be responsible for investment of the capital and any undistributed reserves.

Article 4
Prize

The Sasakawa Health Prize shall consist of a statuette and a sum of money of the order of US$ 100 000 to be given to a person or persons, an institution or institutions, or a nongovernmental organization or organizations having accomplished outstanding innovative work in health development, such as the promotion of given health programmes or notable advances in primary health care, in order to encourage the further development of such work. Current and former staff members of the World Health Organization, and current members of the Executive Board, shall be ineligible to receive the Prize. The sum of money, derived from the income and/or the undistributed reserves, shall be determined by the Prize Selection Panel. The Prize shall be presented during a meeting of the World Health Assembly to the recipient(s) or to a person(s) representing the recipient(s).

Article 5
Prize Selection Panel

The Selection Panel entitled the "Sasakawa Health Prize Selection Panel" shall be composed of: the Chairman of the Executive Board, a member elected by the Executive Board from among its members for a period that may not exceed the duration of his or her terms of office on the Executive Board, and a representative appointed by the Founder.

Article 6
Proposal and selection of candidates for the Prize

Any national health administration as well as any former recipient of the Prize may put forward the name of a candidate for the Prize. Proposals shall be made to the Administrator who will submit them to the Prize Selection Panel together with his technical comments. The Selection Panel will decide in private meeting, by a majority of its members, on the recommendation to be made to the Executive Board of the World Health Organization, whose decision shall be final.

Article 7
Administrator

The Prize shall be administered by its Administrator, namely the Director-General of the World Health Organization, who shall act as Secretary of the Prize Selection Panel.

The Administrator shall be responsible:

1. For the execution of the decisions taken by the Prize Selection Panel within the limits of its powers as defined in these Statutes; and

2. For the observance of the present Statutes and generally for the administration of the Sasakawa Health Prize in accordance with these Statutes.

Article 8
Accountability

Reports on work carried out by recipients of the Prize shall, where appropriate, be submitted annually to the Administrator, who shall be accountable to the World Health Assembly for operations effected by virtue of these Statutes.

Article 9
Revision of the Statutes

On the motion of one of its members, the Prize Selection Panel may propose revision of the present Statutes. Any such motion, if endorsed by a majority of the members of the Selection Panel, shall be submitted to the Executive Board for its approval. Any revision shall be reported for information to the next session of the World Health Assembly.

Annex 2

Sasakawa Health Prize Guidelines (as amended in January 1998)

(1) The Sasakawa Health Prize consisting of a statuette and a sum of money of the order of US$100000, will be awarded for outstanding innovative work in health development.

(2) The Prize will be given to a person or persons, an institution or institutions, or a nongovernmental organization or organizations having accomplished notable advances in the health field in recent years, particularly since the promotion of the strategy for achieving health for all by the year 2000.

(3) The Prize aims at encouraging the further development of outstanding innovative work in health development that has already been accomplished and extends far beyond the call of normal duties; it is not intended as a reward for excellent performance by a candidate of duties normally expected of an official occupying a government position or of a governmental or intergovernmental institution.

(4) The following criteria will be applied in the assessment of the work done by the candidate/candidates:

- **(a)** Contribution to the successful formulation and implementation of the national policy and strategy for health for all by the year 2000;

- **(b)** Promotion of and substantial achievement in advancing given health programmes which have resulted in increasing primary health care coverage, and/or improving the quality of health care to the population, and a notable reduction of given health problems;

- **(c)** Contribution to increased efficiency and management of health systems; policy development, health legislation and ethics, within the framework of primary health care;

- **(d)** Innovative programmes to reach socially and geographically disadvantaged population groups;

- **(e)** Innovative efforts in training and education of health workers in primary health care;

(f) Successful and effective efforts in involving communities in planning, management and evaluation of primary health care programmes;

(g) Development and successful application of health systems research for the advancement of primary health care.

(5) The candidate/candidates nominated for the Prize must be intimately and directly connected with the efforts and achievements in a given area and must have the possibility of remaining involved in the further development of this work.

(6) As one of the main objectives of the Prize is to encourage the further development of such work, the candidate/candidates will be requested to indicate how the award funds would be used for this purpose. The recipient/recipients of the award will, where appropriate, be required to submit annually a report on work carried out to the Administrator of the Prize.

(7) To facilitate the assessment of the work done and the accomplishments, the most recent and pertinent documentation directly related to the work should be submitted along with the nomination. Such materials should illustrate clearly the nature of work carried out, the results achieved, the difficulties and obstacles encountered, and the solutions proposed and implemented; they need not necessarily have been published in a scientific or other journal. Inadequate or inappropriate documentary evidence of the work carried out will greatly handicap the Prize Selection Panel in the assessment of the candidature.

(8) To further support the documentary evidence, if necessary, the Administrator, on behalf of the Prize Selection Panel, reserves the right to examine the work done by the candidate/candidates.

(9) Current and former staff members of the World Health Organization, and current members of the Executive Board, shall be ineligible to receive the Prize.

(10) If more than one candidate is considered eligible by the Prize Selection Panel and selected to receive the Prize, the sum will be proportionately distributed between them.

(11) These guidelines will be reviewed and updated periodically as considered appropriate.

Annex 3

Recipients of the Sasakawa Health Prize

2012
Syamsi Dhuha Foundation (Indonesia)

2011
Dr Eva Siracká (Slovakia)

Pequeña Familia de María/Albergue Maria Association (Panama)

2010
Dr Xueping Du (China)

2009
Dr Amal Abdurrahman Al Jowder (Bahrain)

2008
Movement for Reintegration of People Affected by Hansen's Disease (MORHAN) (Brazil)

2007
Dr Jose Antonio Socrates (Philippines)

2006
International Leprosy Union (India)

Agape Rural Health Program - Holistic Community Based Health Development Program (Puerto Princesa City, Palawan, Philippines)

2005
Centre for Training and Education in Ecology and Health for Peasants (Mexico)

2004
The Family Planning Association of Sri Lanka (Sri Lanka)

2003
Department of Health Center for Health Development - Eastern Visayas (Philippines)

Yemen Leprosy Elimination Society (Republic of Yemen)

2002
Programa Nacional de Atención Odontológica Integral para Mujeres Travbajadoras de Escasos Recursos (Chile)

2001
Dr João Aprigio Guerra de Almeida (Brazil)

2000
Dr Yoav Horn (Israel)

Dr Oviemo Otu Ovadje (Nigeria)

Family Planning Association (PLAFAM) (Venezuela)

1999
Dr J.G. Ortiz Guier (Costa Rica)

Institute of Urban Primary Health Care (South Africa)

1998
Ms Roselyn Mokgantsho Mazibuko (South Africa)

Dr Ahmed Abdul Qadr Al Ghassani (Oman)

Gondar College of Medical Sciences (Ethiopia)

1997
The Mongar Health Services Development Project (Bhutan)

1996
Father A. Gherardi (Chad)

Society for Health Education (Maldives)

1995
Dr J. Torres Goitia Torres (Bolivia)

Professor Le Kinh Due (Viet Nam)

1994
Dr Mo-Im Kim (Republic of Korea)

1993
Professor Oladapo Alabi Ladipo and Mrs Grace Ebun Delano (Nigeria)

Arpana Research and Charities Trust (India)

1992

Dr Handojo Tjandrakusuma (Indonesia)

Mme Brigitte Girault et M. Badara Samb (Senegal)

Canadian Public Health Association (Canada)

1991

Dr Hector Martinez Gomez and Dr Edgar Rey Sanabria (Colombia)

The Regional Centre for Development and Health/Primary Health Care (Benin)

The Vulowai Health Committee (Fiji)

1990

Monsignor Fiorenzo Angelini (Holy See)

Professor B. N. Tandon (India)

Biankouri Health Centre (Togo)

1989

Dr Niu Dongping (China)

1988

Dr Christian Aurenche (France/Cameroon)

Indonesian Family Welfare Movement (PKK) (Indonesia)

1987

Sister Marie Joan Winch (Australia)

1986

Ayadaw Township People's Health Plan Committee (Myanmar)

Dr Lucille Teasdale Corti and Dr Pietro Corti (Uganda)

Dr Amorn Nondasuta (Thailand)

1985

Dr Jesus C. Azurin (Philippines)

Dr David Bersh Escobar (Colombia)

SEWA-RURAL (Society for Education, Welfare and Action - Rural) (India)